Essential Midwifery Practice:
Public Health

Essential Midwifery Practice: Public Health

Edited by

Grace Edwards
RGN, RM, ADM, Cert Ed, MEd, PhD

Sheena Byrom
RGN, RM, MA

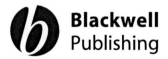

Registered office
John Wiley & Sons Ltd, The Atrium, Southern Gate, Chichester, West Sussex,
PO19 8SQ, United Kingdom

Editorial office
9600 Garsington Road, Oxford, OX4 2DQ, United Kingdom

For details of our global editorial offices, for customer services and for information about
how to apply for permission to reuse the copyright material in this book
please see our website at www.wiley.com/wiley-blackwell.

Library of Congress Cataloging-in-Publication Data
Essential midwifery practice. Public health /
edited by Grace Edwards and Sheena Byrom.
p. ; cm.
Includes bibliographical references and index.
ISBN-13: 978-1-4051-4441-4 (pbk. : alk. paper)
ISBN-10: 1-4051-4441-6 (pbk. : alk. paper)   1. Midwifery — Great Britain.
2. Maternal health services — Great Britain.   I. Edwards, Grace, RN.
II. Byrom, Sheena.   III. Title: Public health.
[DNLM: 1. Midwifery.   2. Maternal Health Services.   3. Maternal Welfare.
4. Nurse's Role.   5. Public Health. WQ 160 E78 2007]

RG950.E66 2007
618.2 — dc22
2006037249

A catalogue record for this book is available from the British Library.

Set in 10/12.5pt Palatino by Graphicraft Ltd, Hong Kong

2   2008

Contents

Preface

Public health is emerging as one of the most important drivers in midwifery, and yet there are few textbooks that address the midwife's role in public health.

This book summarises the important developments in public health over recent years and will relate the recommendations to midwifery practice in a clear and easily understood manner. It highlights issues around health inequalities pertinent to maternity services and promotes individualised, non-judgmental approaches to care.

Integral to this book is the focus on developing a public health philosophy that underpins the role of the midwife. Particular attention is made to the importance of the mother–midwife relationship in maximising the health of the mother and her baby.

Debbie Garrod and **Sheena Byrom** set the scene for the book by critically evaluating medical and social models of maternity care in Chapter 1. The public health agenda is debated in relation to midwifery practice. The strengths and weaknesses of several approaches to care are explored and illustrated by examples of practice. In addition, the role of the midwife as a key component in the social model of care is discussed.

Eileen Stringer builds on Chapter 1 and clearly describes government policy and initiatives related to midwifery. Eileen examines the background to the midwifery public health agenda and explores how the wider determinants of health may impinge on pregnancy and infancy. Practical examples are discussed, for example, how to assess the needs of the community, the use of health equity audits, engaging the community, and the transition from Sure Start to Children's Centres. The midwife's role in public health strategy is explored in depth.

Smoking in pregnancy is a concern for midwives – some may feel ill equipped to support or advise women without appearing judgmental. The chapter by **Grace Edwards** and **David King** describes the prevalence of smoking in pregnancy and explores the issues of tobacco as an addiction. Links between smoking and social class and smoking and breastfeeding are discussed in addition to the effects of smoking on reproduction and child health. The psychology of smoking behaviour is explored, including the use of the cycle of change and motivational theory. Finally, effective smoking cessation strategies and the midwife's role in smoking cessation are highlighted.

Teenage pregnancy in the UK is among the highest in Europe and features as a major concern for the government. **Vanessa Hollings, Claire Jackson** and **Clare McCann** outline the changes in the incidence of teenage pregnancy over several decades, and the effects of being a pregnant teenager are described. There are some suggestions in relation to maternity service provision for this client group with particular attention to engaging with young fathers, and the authors provide an insight into the commissioning cycle and how midwives can influence the process.

Sexual health is another growing concern within public health and is a key driver for the government's white paper *Choosing Health*. **Julie Kelly** and **Grace Edwards** describe the historical trends in sexual health, the recent trends in sexual activity, particularly among young people, and offset the trends in the United Kingdom against the international perspective. The commonest sexually transmitted infections are explained and the current prevalence, consequences and treatment are explored. The psychology of attitudes around sexual health and behaviour is discussed, and advice is given for midwives on offering support and signposting for encouraging a healthy approach to sexual health.

Women who misuse substances present further concerns for midwives. **Lyn McIver** discusses the historical antecedents of substance abuse, and the extent of the problem today. The effects of alcohol and drugs in pregnancy are highlighted in this chapter, and the effects these may have on vulnerable groups are discussed. There are suggestions of how vulnerable families may be supported and the potential adverse effects on future generations should these strategies not be implemented. A holistic approach to caring for women and their families using national models of care concludes this chapter.

Sally Price comprehensively describes the extent of domestic abuse. Sally sensitively discusses the psychology of abuse and the effects this may have on pregnancy. Risk factors and prevalence are explored, along with the role of the midwife in addressing attitudes and myths. The wider effects of domestic abuse on society are also discussed, as well as the role midwives can play in supporting women who disclose domestic abuse.

Another perceived taboo topic is maternal mental health. Women often have difficulty in talking about mental health issues and midwives may feel ill equipped to support and signpost women to appropriate services. **Kathryn Gutteridge, Samuel Dearman** and **Waquas Waheed** outline the issues around maternal mental health and discuss how women's mental health is pivotal to society and family life. The authors explore social perceptions and how to break down barriers to addressing mental health issues. Ways of supporting women with mental health problems are highlighted, supported with case histories. Outlines of the types of mental illness a midwife may encounter are highlighted and the associated stereotypes and stigmas critically explored. Ways in which midwives may support women and promote mental health conclude the chapter.

Chapter 9 describes the practicalities of supporting breast-feeding women using an innovative community model. **Sue Henry, Fiona Dykes, Sheena Byrom, Michelle Atkin** and **Elaine Jackson** give a wider perspective of the global issues and politics that surround breastfeeding. The authors discuss how societal and cultural influences can affect the success of breastfeeding. The politics of breastfeeding are addressed and practical ways of implementing successful breastfeeding strategies discussed. The steps to successful initiation of the Little Angels community breastfeeding business will give hope to midwives who are struggling to support breastfeeding women. It is encouraging to read the accounts from local women themselves and have some insight into their own empowerment.

Soo Downe and **Denis Walsh** present the implications of birth within the wider public health agenda. The authors propose in-depth reasons why midwives consider 'well-being' as part of a social model of childbirth which is based on the concepts of unique normality, salutogenesis, complexity and uncertainty. Clinical examples are used to illustrate how positive experiences can impinge on the wider perspectives of a woman's life and that of her family.

We are excited and proud to be able to present this important and timely book that we hope will inform, educate and promote an understanding of how public health should underpin the work of every midwife.

Grace Edwards and Sheena Byrom
January 2007

Foreword

It is a pleasure to write a Foreword to this timely and important book. More than ever, it is essential that midwives understand their pivotal and life-enhancing role in public health as well as the many unexploited opportunities to improve the quality of life and health of some of our more vulnerable sections of society. With knowledge comes power, and with power the ability to change the lives of childbearing women and their families for the better.

The chapters set out in this book mirror the public health and policy agenda in all four countries of the UK in 2006–2007. Smoking, sexual health, substance abuse, domestic abuse and – probably most importantly – poverty, continue to be the major public health issues of the first decade of the 21st century. Even in the affluent 21st century, poverty and ill health remain major and contentious issues.

In 2003 Professor Sir Liam Donaldson delivered his independent report to government on aspects of the nation's health. He reviewed progress in what he called '*a longstanding problem of health inequalities*'. He reaffirmed that there was still a large gap in the standards of health between people in affluent sections of society and those in the most disadvantaged. He showed how in some communities death rates were comparable with the national average in the 1950s. He demonstrated the North–South (of England) divide, with people living in the North being much worse off in terms of health. He wrote:

> Health inequalities have lasted hundreds of years or more. There is little sign that they are narrowing and in some fields the gap between social groups seems actually to be widening . . . sustained commitment is essential and progress should be rigorously audited and reported publicly . . . reducing health inequalities

is a long-term task but maintaining it as a priority for government as well as statutory and other agencies is vitally important

So we do have a problem, it's official.

In 2003–2004 12.3 million people living in the UK were poor, living
in households with below 60% of median income after housing
costs. In 2003–2004 28% of children (that is 3.5 million) were still
living in poverty. Children from manual social backgrounds are
still 1$\frac{1}{2}$ times more likely to die as infants than children from non-
manual social backgrounds. Children in social class V are still five
times more likely to die in an accident than those in social class I,
and babies from manual social backgrounds are still 1$\frac{1}{4}$ times
more likely to be of low birthweight than those from non-manual
social backgrounds.

Teenage motherhood is eight times as common among those
from manual social backgrounds as for those from professional
backgrounds, and five-year-olds in Wales and Scotland have, on
average, more than twice as many missing, decayed or filled teeth
as five-year-olds in the West Midlands and South-East.

According to the charity Shelter:

> Every day in Britain, more than one million children wake up in
> squalid, temporary or crowded accommodation – bad housing
> is making our children ill, robbing them of a decent education
> and damaging their future

What an indictment of nearly sixty years of a welfare state with
health care still free at the 'point of delivery' in 2007. We have an
unequal society and midwives are privileged to provide care on
the front line: they are there with women. They are there when
others have left and are safely in their offices away from the problems
that beset women and their families. Midwives have the unique
opportunity to develop a therapeutic relationship with women at a
time when they may be more inclined to listen. Not only do childbearing women have their own interests at heart but they also have
the interests of their unborn child and new family to consider. This
presents midwives with an opportunity not to be missed.

This book will help midwives in clinical practice (and in education too) to understand the complexities of the public health policy
and practice agenda. The reader will learn that there are no quick
fixes and that judgmental care is not caring or helpful. It will also
help the reader to unravel the social context of many of the difficulties that can undermine childbearing women as they struggle to
make sense of their lives.

I hope this book will help all midwives to see that women are often not so much disadvantaged by poverty, drug and substance abuse, race, disability, sexual orientation, or even unplanned pregnancy, but they *can* be disadvantaged by the inappropriate attitudes of those who offer them care and support. It is only by understanding the complexities involved in improving health that we can sensitively and compassionately help those who need us the most.

I think the editors and contributors have made a significant contribution to improving the state of the nation's health and I commend this book to midwives, educators, students and all who are challenged by the inequalities in British society in the 21st century.

Professor Sheila C Hunt
Dundee August 2006

On the state of the public health: Annual report of the Chief Medical Officer 2003

Annual report. Donaldson, Liam; Department of Health 28/07/2004 Department of Health Crown

http://england.shelter.org.uk/home/index.cfm accessed August 2 2006

Notes on the Contributors

Michelle Atkin BA (Hons) is a mother to six children, and passionate about breastfeeding, especially protecting and promoting. She is one of the directors of Little Angels breastfeeding support, a funded project unique in that it employs local mothers from the community to support breastfeeding mothers. All breastfeeding mothers within a defined area are seen and offered support. Her passion is to make breastfeeding fashionable; to challenge and change society's perception and view of breastfeeding; and to make it the norm.

Sheena Byrom RN, RM, MA is a consultant midwife and has a joint appointment with East Lancashire Hospitals NHS Trust and the University of Central Lancashire. Sheena has worked as a midwife for 28 years in various roles including a GP maternity unit, consultant unit and in the community. Sheena's interests include addressing the consequences of health inequalities through the development of targeted services for those most in need. She has published in midwifery journals and has presented nationally and internationally on this subject.

Samuel Dearman is training to be a psychiatrist. He is a graduate from the University of Manchester and continues to study there as a postgraduate research student. Sam has been involved in research in psychiatry since before graduating as a doctor and regularly publishes articles in peer-reviewed journals. Sam's research interests include liaison psychiatry, mental health legislation and evidenced-based service provision.

Professor Soo Downe BA (Hons), RM, MSc, PhD spent 15 years working in various clinical, research, and project development roles at Derby City General Hospital. From January 2001, Soo has worked at the University of Central Lancashire (UCLAN) in England, where she is now the professor of midwifery studies. She set up the UCLAN Women's, Infant, and Sexual Health (WISH) Institute, which was launched in October 2002. She currently chairs the UK Royal College of Midwives Campaign for Birth steering committee. Her main research focus at present is the nature of, and culture around, normal birth, and she is the editor of *Normal Childbirth: evidence and debate*, which has sold well internationally since its publication in 2004.

Dr Fiona Clare Dykes PhD, MA, Cert Ed, ADM, RM, RGN is reader in maternal and infant health and leads the Maternal and Infant Nutrition and Nurture Unit (MAINN), in the Institute for Women, Infant and Sexual Health, University of Central Lancashire, UK. Fiona has a particular focus upon the social, political and economic influences upon infant feeding practices, globally. Fiona is domain editor for the international journal *Maternal and Child Nutrition*, and has worked on projects funded by WHO, UNICEF, Department of Health and National Institute of Clinical Excellence (NICE). Fiona is co-editor of *Maternal and Infant Nutrition and Nurture: Controversies and Challenges* (Quay books) and author of *Breastfeeding in Hospital: Mothers, Midwives and the Production Line* (Routledge).

Dr Grace Edwards RGN, RM, ADM, Cert Ed, MEd, PhD qualified as a midwife in 1978 and worked as a hospital midwife and a community midwife for 12 years, during which time she completed the Advanced Diploma of Midwifery and the Certificate in Education. She worked as a midwife teacher in 1988 and completed a master's degree in education. In 1993 she took up post as regional co-ordinator for the Confidential Enquiry into Stillbirths and Deaths in Infancy (CESDI) and the Congenital Anomaly Survey, a post she held until 2002. During this time she completed a PhD on People's Perceptions of Healthy Pregnancy. Since 2002 she has been employed as consultant midwife in public health in Liverpool. In 2004 she accepted a post as principal lecturer in midwifery research at the University of Central Lancashire. She is currently working in both roles as a joint appointment. In 2005 she was appointed as national midwifery assessor for the Confidential Enquiry into Maternal and Child Health (CEMACH) for maternal mortality.

Debbie Garrod BA (Hons), MA, PGCE, RM is consultant midwife in public health at Stockport NHS Foundation Trust. Debbie came to midwifery from a background in teaching and training and has been a National Childbirth Trust (NCT) teacher since 1982. In 1993 she completed her preregistration training at Stepping Hill Hospital, Stockport. Following qualification she worked at four different trusts in Greater Manchester in a range of roles, focusing on developing services for vulnerable groups of women. She also spent a year on secondment at Manchester University, returning to Stockport in 2002 to take up her current role.

Kathryn Gutteridge MSc, Dip Counselling and Psychotherapy, SEN, RGN, RM, SoM is consultant midwife working within a public health remit leading on maternal mental health, domestic violence and abuse issues. Kathryn has worked with women with mental health issues during childbirth for over 10 years and has developed services and therapeutic support programmes, which have been recognised as highly effective. She is very motivated to address the stigma that exists in this area and has presented her work nationally and internationally. She has drawn attention to the little known area in childbirth of surviving sexual abuse and the impact it has for the mothering experience. She is co-founder of Sanctum Midwives, a group of midwives who have experienced sexual abuse; raising awareness through research, publication and education. Kathryn is a feminist, a humanist and interested in attachment theory.

Sue Henry RGN, RM, Dip HE (midwifery) is the infant feeding co-ordinator for East Lancashire Hospitals NHS Trust and partner co-ordinator for Little Angels Darwen Ltd. Sue qualified as a midwife 12 years ago, having varied experience in team midwifery. She has specialised in breastfeeding support over the last three years, helping to maintain Baby Friendly Accreditation on one hospital site and working towards the award on another. She has been involved in developing peer support activities in the hospital and in local communities.

Vanessa Hollings MSc, MBA, SRD is deputy director of commissioning with Blackburn with Darwen Primary Care Trust, working in partnership with the Borough Council to develop integrated children's services. She has lead responsibility for the commissioning of children's services for children and young people aged 0–19 years and has an overall role as lead for children's services across the PCT. As well as the commissioning role, Vanessa manages a youth health team, a successful healthy living centre initiative and was instrumental in the development of the Blackburn West

Sure Start scheme. Vanessa has wide experience of health service provision, both in a hospital and community setting, and partnership working – as a paediatric dietitian in Cambridgeshire and community health development manager in Blackburn – before moving into commissioning.

Claire Jackson BSc, MSc (Econ), DMS is the young persons' sexual health strategy co-ordinator with Blackburn with Darwen Primary Care Trust and Borough Council. Claire has worked with young people and sexual health in the voluntary and statutory sector since completing a Masters in Population Policies and Programmes in 1998. Claire enjoys the challenge of bringing agencies to work together and developing the best possible sexual health education, information and services, and empowering pregnant teenagers and young parents to access services that meet their specific needs.

Elaine Jackson (FPC) is mother of two children and breastfed them both, her youngest to three years. She is one of the directors of Little Angels Darwen Ltd breastfeeding support, a funded project unique in that it employs local mothers from the community to support breastfeeding mothers.

Julie Kelly BA (Hons), MPH is an experienced senior public health specialist who has worked in the health service for almost 10 years. Her portfolios and areas of responsibility have been diverse and they include sexual health, cervical screening, support for teenage parents, breast screening and performance management. Julie has worked at the local and regional level and some of her previous posts include teenage pregnancy and parenting lead for Liverpool and north-west regional sexual health lead. She is currently based in Liverpool PCT where she works as a public health specialist leading on sexual health.

David King MSc undertook his first degree at Hope University where he studied biology and sport. He obtained an MSc in 2003 during which he combined his interest in sport with health issues by undertaking a study into physical activity behaviour in middle-aged women. He has previously worked for the Centre for Health research and Evaluation based at Edge Hill University, researching health-related issues. In 2005 he took up post as a research assistant at the University of Central Lancashire to investigate smoking cessation in pregnancy (the SCIP study).

Clare McCann MSc is the public health partnerships manager for Blackburn with Darwen Borough Council and Primary Care Trust. Clare has a background in youth and community work and has experience of working for voluntary and statutory organisations, in the UK and abroad. Clare's experience of working with girls and young women led to her post as teenage pregnancy strategy co-ordinator, during which time she completed a master's degree in applied public health.

Lyn McIver qualified as a nurse in 1978 and practised for most of her professional life as a neonatal nurse/specialist nurse in Liverpool maternity services. An interest in pregnant women who use drugs and the effects on the baby led her to undertake a master's degree. Lyn graduated from Liverpool John Moores University in 1997. Published papers include 'Identification of neonatal abstinence syndrome after maternal methadone therapy' in the *Archive of Diseases in Childhood* (1994). Lyn works in a strategic role as lead commissioner representing health, local authority, probation and the police in interpreting the national drugs policy and the local delivery across the city of Liverpool.

Sally Price registered as a midwife in 1993, since when she has worked in all areas of the maternity service, and became a supervisor of midwives in 2000. In November 2000, Sally was appointed to her current role as a consultant midwife. Sally is a nationally recognised expert in the field of domestic abuse. For the past six years she has led a training programme that prepares midwives and other health professionals to handle domestic violence issues. She was a researcher involved in a Department of Health funded research project 'An impact evaluation of an education and support programme to promote the introduction of routine antenatal enquiry for domestic violence' at North Bristol NHS Trust. She is co-author of a commissioned domestic violence training pack and video. Sally is also a member of the National Domestic Violence and Health Research Forum.

Eileen Stringer RN, RM, DPSM, SoM, BSc(Hons), MPH is a consultant midwife in public health for the Pennine Acute Hospitals Trust, which includes four maternity units with nearly 10 500 deliveries per year. Eileen qualified as a midwife in 1984 and has held both clinical and managerial roles, including labour ward and community midwifery, with time spent as a senior midwife practitioner and deputy head of midwifery. Eileen's career focus for the last 10 years has been to promote a public health approach to maternity services, particularly in the community setting. For the last three years, her current role has led to close working relationships with PCTs, local authorities and voluntary organisations linked to the trust.

Dr Waquas Waheed MBBS, MRCPsych is a consultant psychiatrist in crisis resolution and home treatment team in Lancashire, UK. He qualified from Pakistan and was trained in Pakistan, Coventry and later in Manchester, UK in general adult and liaison psychiatry. Waquas is actively involved in research and focuses on depression, self-harm and suicide in women particularly in ethnic minorities. His ongoing work includes developing and successfully testing a social group intervention for depressed ethnic minority women. He regularly publishes in peer-reviewed journals and has contributed chapters to a number of books. At the University of Manchester he lectures on postgraduate courses and supervises research degrees.

Denis Walsh RM, RGN, DPSM, PGDipEd, MA, PhD is senior lecturer in research at the University of Central Lancashire and an independent midwifery consultant, teaching on evidence and normal birth. Denis trained as a midwife in Leicester, UK and has worked in a variety of midwifery environments. He publishes widely on normal birth.

Acknowledgements

We would like to thank all the chapter authors for their sterling work in completing these chapters, especially those who had personal issues to deal with at the same time.

Acknowledgements and special thanks to the Little Angels breastfeeding supporters, who told their stories for Chapter 9. At their request, pseudonyms have been used. They are Louise Dunn, Shahnaz Abdullah, Louise Elarkham, Clare Bradley, Aisha Ahmed, Nazra Khan, Qubra Ali, Kirsty Hymers, Lisa Clarke, Marie Goulding and Fiona Eaton.

From Waquas Waheed and Samuel Dearman, thanks to Mrs Vivienne Walker and Mrs Jackie Turnbull of the Lantern Centre Library, Lancashire Care NHS Trust for their support and patience throughout the writing of Chapter 8.

Finally we would both like to thank our husbands Robin and Paul – they know why!!

Grace Edwards and Sheena Byrom
January 2007

Chapter 1
The Midwifery Public Health Agenda: Setting the Scene

Debbie Garrod and Sheena Byrom

> If you wish to foretell the health of future generations, look in the perambulators
>
> (Nye Bevan, at the inauguration of the National Health Service (NHS) in 1948)

What is public health?

> Public health aims to address the health and healthcare needs of populations, bringing together all the factors which shape and influence the health of individuals and communities
>
> (Royal College of Midwives (RCM) 2001)

Public health seeks to protect and improve the health of communities: it works to identify the underlying causes of health and well-being, and also of disease and ill health, looking for patterns and trends in particular populations. Public health sets health in its widest social and political context. It draws direct links, for example, between factors such as levels of employment, standards of housing, educational attainment and concomitant levels of health and ill health, which are described fully in Chapter 2. It uses the evidence on these links to develop social policy aimed to have a positive impact on the wider determinants of health (RCM 2001).

The purpose of this book is to increase midwives' knowledge base on a whole range of public health issues that have a direct impact on the health and well-being of the families in their care. Pregnancy is unique in giving a window of opportunity for making changes in lifestyle and habits. At no other time in life do people have such regular contact with health professionals, and this book aims to help midwives to maximise this opportunity for health gain. The special challenge for midwives is to achieve and maintain the appropriate balance between addressing the needs of 'populations' and meeting the individual needs of every woman and her family.

Public health populations

The term 'population' deserves defining in the context of public health with particular reference to midwifery and three examples are described below (Department of Health (DoH) 1999a).

Geographical

A population may be geographical. For example, living on a housing estate with particular needs and problems will have clear implications for the health and well-being of young families. These problems may include, for instance, street crime, lack of shopping and leisure facilities, poor public transport and inadequate health services – a dearth of dentists, for example. The geographical location of this housing estate will put multiple barriers and challenges in the path of young parents who are striving to give their baby the best possible start in life.

Client groups

A further example of a population is an identified client group. In public health terms, there is no 'one-size-fits-all' approach to maternity care. Rather, the particular needs of specified client groups are identified, and special measures taken to design care to meet the needs of this group. Examples of populations identified by client group include teenage parents, asylum-seeking families and travelling communities. When developing appropriate services for such groups of women, maternity services will work in close liaison with a wide range of agencies, for example, housing, benefits and education. This close interagency working characterises the public health approach to midwifery care.

Particular health needs

A population may consist of a group of people with a particular health need, which may or may not have existed before the pregnancy. Women with mental health problems, for example, have a particular set of needs during the childbearing continuum, as do women with diabetes. As with the previous example of a population (a specified client group), midwives will be involved in working in collaboration with other agencies and disciplines, ensuring effective communication and care planning for each woman.

In working with these different 'populations' of women, taking a public health approach to midwifery enables women and their families to use pregnancy as a time of unique opportunity for improving health and well-being and reducing inequalities in health. Thus midwives begin to realise their potential as public health practitioners, whose

> key role . . . is to identify and influence those factors which promote the health of the population
>
> (DoH 1999b)

In the framework of public health 'populations', midwives should hold at the heart of their practice that in every situation, the group or 'population' is made up of individual women and families. A public health approach to midwifery care requires that midwives at all times maintain a balance in their perspective – between awareness of the shared needs of the population and the special and individual needs of the woman and the family for whom she is caring.

On the level of the individual, there is ample evidence that what happens during preconception, pregnancy, labour, birth and the early years of life has a lasting impact on the individual's health. A poor start in life will have a negative impact on the health and well-being of that person for the rest of his or her life. The effects of poverty and deprivation are perpetuated through generations, creating a downward spiral of chronic ill health and premature death in families and communities. For instance, a mother on a low income who is unable to afford an adequate diet in pregnancy is more likely to give birth to an undernourished baby. This baby in turn is more likely to suffer from coronary heart disease, stroke and non-insulin dependent diabetes in later life (Barker and Clark 1997). A public health approach to midwifery enables midwives to use the knowledge and evidence that exists about trends and patterns of wellness and disease; and to offer personalised and appropriate care to address these needs.

What does your local community look like?

When striving to provide individualised, appropriate, family-centred care, midwives and health care workers must think about the women and families they care for, where they live, their social and cultural backgrounds. If care is to be appropriate and effective, there needs to be an assessment at a community and individual level. Some aspects of needs assessment are addressed in Chapter 2. These include signposting to relevant toolkits and policy documents.

Health needs assessment is a systematic method for reviewing the health issues facing a population, which informs policy and sets priorities for appropriate resources to improve health and reduce inequalities (Health Development Agency (HDA) 2005). To be concise, it presents an opportunity to engage with local communities, other healthcare providers and commissioners, and provides the evidence to plan appropriate services, targeted at those most in need. *Every Child Matters* (Department for Education and Skills (DfES) 2004) highlighted the necessity of a shared assessment of local needs for children, young people and their families, including the involvement of this client group. The paper also stresses the importance of accurate information, and honesty in relation to how well local children and young people are already supported and what the key challenges are.

What can midwives do?

Initiate a small piece of research into an area that you work in, examining the demographics and social status of the families who live there.

- Think about the women and families you serve: are they well informed and accessing services? If not, how can you improve their access to information and choice?
- Look at your team statistics, for example, examine babies' birthweights in your caseload. Then ask your team to help you find out a little more about those data. Do they relate to access to services, culture or midwifery practice?
- Carry out a small survey to find out what women like in relation to an area of service provision, for example, postnatal visits.
- Be creative and think differently about how you care for women. Use opportunities to change the way you provide care, for example, Children's Centres and postnatal 'drop-in' sessions. Discuss your ideas with your managers and develop a plan.

Case study: population

Women from black and minority ethnic backgrounds living in the UK are at increased risk of inequalities in access to maternity services, with limited communication (Neile 1997, Maternity Alliance 2004). Evidence is clear that some babies are at greater risk of mortality dependent on their mother's place of birth. South Asian heritage populations are also at increased risk of Type 2 diabetes (Burden *et al.* 2000).

Shazia was born in Pakistan, and doesn't speak English. She came to the north-west of England to be married, and is now pregnant with her first child. She attends all her antenatal sessions, but doesn't know what will happen to her body when she goes into labour, apart from the little her mother told her before she came to England. She was informed recently that she had gestational diabetes, and didn't really understand what that meant. She would like to attend the drop-in sessions the midwives run, but feels nervous. Most days she feels sad, but doesn't know why. Moreover, she can't tell anyone that she feels sad, for many reasons.

And what about her baby?

Figure 1.1 demonstrates the increased risks for Shazia's baby. Midwives can use this evidence and local data to influence or change service provision.

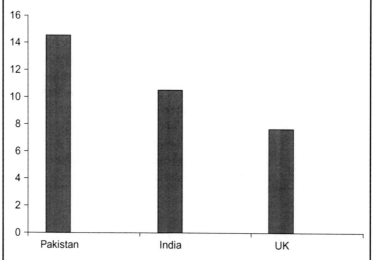

Figure 1.1 Perinatal mortality rates 2002, linked by mother's country of birth.
Source: Office for National Statistics (2002).

Examples of good practice: developing your idea (1)

- A midwife working in the antenatal clinic at the hospital noticed that many of the women who attended the medical clinic with gestational diabetes were from South Asian heritage communities.
- She asked the audit department in her unit to help her to analyse the figures so she had the exact number.
- She shared her findings with colleagues and asked for help in developing a plan to improve services for the women attending.
- The proposal included doing a literature search to present as a background, thereby informing and strengthening the local data.
- Women with gestational diabetes were involved in planning the new service, with particular attention given to those who did not speak English.
- Local women helped and became involved (as volunteers) in setting up and delivering nutrition awareness sessions in the clinic waiting room.

Examples of good practice: developing your idea (2)

- A team of midwives working in a deprived area with high unemployment rates and a 99% Caucasian population, noticed that a small group of asylum-seeking families had recently moved to the area.
- The families were isolated by a broad range of factors, including their ethnicity, language and asylum-seeking status.
- They did not know what health services were available – or how to access them. Some women thought they had to pay for maternity care, or for aspects of it – having an epidural, for example.
- The midwives talked to the families about their needs and brought together a range of agencies (housing, welfare rights, support group for asylum seekers) and pooled knowledge.
- Together, they devised a 'map' to signpost how to access the whole range of support services available for asylum-seeking families. They gave this to all midwives in the organisation to help them give better and more appropriate care.

Avoidance of stigmatisation

Although understanding populations is important, it is crucial that midwives avoid placing 'labels' on populations, and thus treating them uniformly in a defined group. For example, not all teenage parents are vulnerable and unsupported, and some women who misuse drugs are able to remain in employment and successfully care for their family. Although this book has divided certain populations into specific chapters, the main focus is the underpinning uniqueness of each individual woman.

Hunt (2004) has written extensively about the effects of poverty on women using maternity services. She describes the governmental response to addressing population health as 'structural' solutions to poverty. The 'structures' are defined as policy documents, for example *Saving Lives: Our Healthier Nation* (DoH 1999a) and programmes of support such as Sure Start local programmes and the Teenage Pregnancy Unit. Structural solutions are described in more detail below. Hunt's work (2004) demonstrates the importance of these approaches, but reinforces the potential of the unique relationship between midwife and woman on an 'individual' level. The midwife–mother relationship is described in more detail later in this chapter.

This book sets birth as a social, psychological and biological event. It builds on Hunt's work by demonstrating how an 'individual' positive relationship between woman and midwife during any part of the childbirth experience has the potential to maximise health outcomes for mother and baby.

Background to the midwifery public health agenda

A brief review of the professionalisation of midwifery illustrates that it has its roots firmly embedded in public health. In the late 1880s, The Midwives Institute (a group of middle-class philanthropic women) began a two-pronged campaign: for the training and practice of midwives to be regulated; and to ensure that all women had access to the services of a midwife for the birth of their babies. Both these aspirations are closely aligned to public health principles. Their work led to the passing of the first Midwives' Act in 1902. Before the passing of the Midwives' Act, most women (85%) delivered their babies at home. The majority of women were attended by a 'handywoman' who was not a health professional but a 'traditional birth attendant', qualified by her own life experience and her age. There was very little in the way of systematic 'preventative antenatal care' until the 1920s and 30s, following the Maternal and Child Welfare Act of 1918 (Leap and Hunter 1993:159).

During the 1930s, a National Maternity Service was established with the aim of making childbearing safer by improving existing services, based on free domiciliary midwifery care. The services were provided through local authority public health departments. Trained midwives offered basic antenatal and postnatal as well as intrapartum care; there were systems established for referral to general practitioners (GPs) or other specialist services (Peretz 1990). Midwives were employed by these local authority public health departments until as recently as 1974, when they moved into the employ of the NHS.

The provision of universally accessible maternity care under the auspices of the NHS, following its inauguration in 1948, follows one of the basic and underlying principles of public health practice. That is, the provision of free and comprehensive maternity services provided largely by community-based midwives, whose role included health promotion and education about nutrition and hygiene. Indeed it is documented that on occasion midwives would take meals to homes they were visiting (Leap and Hunter 1993).

Midwives and public health

Midwives have always been public health practitioners, as defined by the activities in which they are involved. The Royal College of Midwives (RCM 2001), in a position paper *The Midwife's Role in Public Health* outlined the public health activities that all midwives are involved in when providing midwifery care to individual and groups of women. For example, midwives offer information and advice on a broad range of issues, including healthy eating, exercise, screening tests, support to stop smoking and promotion of breastfeeding. Birth is a public health issue because of its impact on the health and well-being of women, babies, children, families and society (Sandall 2004), and will be explored further in this chapter.

An underlying principle of public health is that it makes its impact 'upstream', aiming to prevent problems before they arise and to promote long-term well-being. An analogy (Ashton and Seymour 1998) is used to demonstrate this upstream thinking by equating health workers to lifesavers standing by a fast-flowing river. Every so often, a drowning person is swept alongside. The lifesaver dives in to the rescue, and retrieves and resuscitates the 'patient'. Just as they have finished, another casualty appears alongside. The lifesavers are so busy that they have no time to walk upstream and think about why so many people are falling in the river.

It could be argued that what is necessary is to refocus upstream, and more 'upstream' thinking amongst health workers. If midwives reflect on the antenatal admissions, and contemplate how much of the care is reactive, they may consider the women who are admitted with poor fetal growth. On an individual level, are there any factors that could have contributed such as race, culture, social environment, life choices and domestic abuse?

How can midwives think differently in delivering antenatal care to prevent low birthweight? Midwives are uniquely placed to deliver health messages in a facilitative supportive manner, as women are more receptive to health messages during pregnancy. Where better to begin than at birth, for as *Making a Difference* clearly states:

> Midwives have contact with people at critical points in their lives, which offer significant opportunities to promote health
>
> (DoH 1999b:60)

Midwives have become increasingly familiar with, and part of the driving force for, the new public health movement since the publication of two key documents in 1999 (DoH 1999a; DoH 1999b). Their involvement in the renaissance and excitement of working in new ways to improve the health of mothers and families was, primarily, in the shadow of other health professionals, until they embraced the challenge to work in Sure Start initiatives and mainstream models of addressing social exclusion. In 2001, the English National Board (ENB 2001) celebrated the achievements of midwives who led public health initiatives and improved maternity services for the vulnerable groups and communities they served. Since that time, there has been a proliferation of public health activity where midwives are key agents in creating and developing a culture of care that addresses the needs of individual women in local populations.

Structural influence on midwifery practice

Socially structured solutions to addressing health inequalities have influenced midwifery practice. The creation of specific public health roles for midwives is an important part of the implementation of Government strategy to tackle the root causes of ill health since the late 1990s. As the profile of the public health agenda has increased, so has the number of midwifery roles with 'public health' in their title, plus 'new' specialist midwifery roles focusing on teenage pregnancy, smoking cessation, domestic violence. Specialist roles have changed the face of midwifery and provided the profession with opportunity to develop and refocus care provision to those with highest needs. The leadership strand to these posts is to 'mainstream' public health thinking – to facilitate a ripple effect throughout maternity services. The overarching aim for specialist roles is to develop pathways of care that enhance core services for hard-to-reach women, so that all midwives are enabled to think differently when providing care. That is, new approaches to care; care based on what women and families need and want.

Public health work at a governmental level, through the publication of White Papers for example, takes a societal perspective, aiming to reduce the inequalities in health. Health and social policy in relation to the inequalities agenda have driven the structural changes throughout the health service, and are described further in Chapter 2. The first Government report to highlight the correlation between poverty and health inequalities was the Black Report in 1982 (HMSO 1980), although the links between social deprivation and ill health and early death have been recognised since philanthropists in early Victorian times worked to improve the lives, homes and health of the poorest members of society. Health policy in response to Sir Donald Acheson's report in 1998 recognises that the cycle of poverty and deprivation, unless broken, perpetuates from generation to generation. The main policy drivers include:

- Black Report (HMSO 1982)
- Acheson Report (DoH 1998)
- *Saving Lives: Our Healthier Nation* (DoH 1999a)
- *The NHS Plan* (DoH 2000)
- *Tackling Health Inequalities* (DoH 2003b)
- Confidential Enquiry into Maternal and Child Health (CEMACH 2004)
- *Every Child Matters* (DfES 2004)
- *Children, Young People and Maternity Services National Service Framework* (DoH 2004a)
- *Choosing Health* (DoH 2004e)
- *Our Health, Our Care, Our Say* (DoH 2006)

The documents have a repetitive theme; they demonstrate the clear picture of the relationship between poverty and ill health. For example:

Women living in the most deprived areas of England had a 45% higher death rate than those living in the most affluent areas

(CEMACH 2004)

What can midwives do?

The above documents provide midwives with the evidence, the tools for change, when wanting to improve services or do things differently. The change may be small but significant, such as working in Children's Centres (outlined in two recent policy drivers DoH 2004b; DoH 2006) or the development of guidelines or care pathways.

Examples of good practice: using policy in practice

Every Child Matters (DfES 2004) gives five priority outcomes for children, and is a key document informing statutory and voluntary health, education and social care organisations. The outcomes are:

- Being healthy
- Staying safe
- Enjoying and achieving
- Making a positive contribution
- Achieving economic well-being

Three midwives used these five outcomes as a framework to develop a care pathway for teenage parents (see Chapter 3).

Another area of positive political influence for UK midwives are public service agreement (PSA) targets, which aim to transform the health and social care system so that it produces faster, fairer services that deliver better health and tackle health inequalities (DoH 2004b). These are the only targets for maternity services, and pursuing goals to achieve them comes with extra funding to pump-prime initiatives.

The targets incorporate the reduction of smoking in pregnancy, reducing teenage pregnancies, and increasing breastfeeding rates; all relevant to midwifery practice. By collaborating with primary care trusts and local authorities, midwives can be part of the planning and development of new initiatives to meet the targets through working differently and with extra resources. See Chapter 3 for an example of how this has been achieved in one area in north-west England.

Public health policy taking the population view has the potential to emerge from a positivist paradigm where statistics and certainty set the agenda. Two key policy drivers for maternity services (DoH 1993; DoH 2004a) have endeavoured to offer an alternative by investigating views of women and stakeholders through qualitative approaches.

Changing Childbirth (DoH 1993) was a significantly important structured response for the midwifery profession. The report stated that the first principle of maternity services should be that 'the woman must be the focus of maternity care', going on to emphasise that 'for every woman, pregnancy and birth are a unique experience'. This marked a significant shift away from the institutionalised and medicalised approach to childbearing that had become the norm in the 1970s and 1980s.

The second guiding principle of *Changing Childbirth* was meeting the needs of the individual. The document clearly stated that services should be 'flexible and responsive to the needs of families being served'. These underlying principles continue to guide the development of services today, as well as the practice of midwives and the education of students. Latterly, the *National Service Framework for Children, Young People and Maternity Services* (DoH 2004a) built on the principles of the *Changing Childbirth* document. Module 11 of the document states that maternity services should be:

> Flexible individualised services designed to fit around the woman and her baby's journey through pregnancy and motherhood, with emphasis on the needs of vulnerable and disadvantaged women
>
> (DoH 2004a:4)

The individualisation of childbirth is a fundamental public health issue, as it sees birth as an event unique to that individual, which maximises the opportunity both for positive birth outcomes and for changes in lifestyle and subsequent long-term health improvements.

Individual midwifery response

Healthcare organisation depends very much on politics, culture and structural forces, but maternity is unique in its implications on the reproduction of society and the promotion of normality (Sandall 2005). Midwives are present before and at the beginning of life, when the scene is set for future health. They are in a key position to influence maternal and perinatal health outcomes, by the very nature of their role. But how midwives 'are' in that role is the key to the promotion of health and well-being.

Midwives must remember that each pregnancy, labour, birth and motherhood is unique. Individualised care is symbolised by a midwife building a relationship with the woman, adapting care appropriately, using their 'radar' – what they see, hear and feel – to assess the woman's needs. This individual approach to care rejects condemnatory attitudes that form barriers to access to care, where women feel they are being judged according to where they live, their colour or life choices.

It is important that midwives try to look beyond the individual encounter with the woman, whether it is at an antenatal appointment, attending her birth, or visiting her after the baby has been born, and try to understand 'where the woman is coming from'. Midwives should try to understand the influences the woman has had in her life that support her chosen path even though detrimental to her and her baby's health, and try not to impose their own personal values on her approach to care. Adopting a public health approach enables midwives to see these 'choices' in the context of all the circumstances that impact on the woman's life: her background, social circumstances, opportunities and aspirations. Wanless (2002) claims that in order to have an influence on prevention of ill health, there must be an understanding of communities and why individuals exhibit symptoms of their societal circumstance.

It could be suggested that individualised care is based on a slight change in the proverb 'do unto others as you would have them do unto you', to 'do unto others as they would have done unto them'. In her book, Hunt (2004) describes how invaluable the midwife's role is in supporting women who are affected by poverty. Hunt's view is clearly demonstrated, as women who have children will usually have a one-to-one relationship with at least one midwife during their childbearing years. Midwives, Hunt goes on to suggest, have a unique opportunity to develop a relationship and listen, hear, notice and respond to women as individuals. In her study into why women chose home births, Edwards (2000) emphasises the importance of a trusting relationship where caregivers support and facilitate the woman through attentive nurturing. The author prompts midwives to 'look below the surface: listen more closely' (Edwards 2000:63), and demonstrates how underlying differences in belief systems affected women's relationships with their midwives in the key areas of support, control, power and trust.

Through individualised care that embraces the understanding of individual societal circumstance, midwives have the opportunity to influence the future of two lives. However, not all women are able to express their wishes, for many reasons. The Changing Childbirth document (1993) was informed from accounts of women who were, on the whole, able to articulate their views. The unheard voices from that time remain largely unheard, of women who feel disempowered or unable to say what they would or would not like in maternity services. Many women may not fully understand the services available to them, let alone the implications of the proposed model of care or intervention. Hunt (2004) is clear that for women living in social exclusion and poverty, their needs are more complex, and she urges midwives to 'see' things differently and to listen to women's views after asking them sensitively what they would like.

Points for reflection: 'unheard' voices

Jane is a middle-class white woman attending her antenatal appointment. Today she hopes to see the obstetrician as she is 36 weeks pregnant and would like to have a vaginal birth following a previous caesarean section for breech presentation. In addition, due to her back problem, she preferred not to be continuously monitored and wanted to know if she could use the birth pool for early labour. The consultant is unavailable, and she is seen by the registrar and midwife who inform her that she would have to be continuously monitored and could not use the pool, as it would contravene the local guideline.

Jane was devastated, not only with the decision, but with the apparent inability of those health professionals to really 'listen' to her. By chance, she personally knew a midwife who helped her to arrange a second opinion, which led to a mutual agreement for Jane's wishes to be met. Primarily, it was Jane's personal contact with a member of staff that enabled her wishes to be considered. But it could be argued that if Jane was unable to speak English for example, or had a history of depression, she would not have received the same opportunity to express her concerns. Indeed, she may not have had any worries about decisions made for her, limiting the 'knowledge' of choice for the privileged few.

The essence of public health midwifery lies in seeking and achieving the delicate balance between focusing on the needs of the individual woman, while taking into account the context in which the woman lives. To meet the full potential of their public health role, midwives must be aware of the needs not only of individual women, but also of their families, communities, and wider populations, as described above.

Social versus medical model of midwifery care

Public health is not an 'add-on' extra to midwifery practice, but an underpinning philosophy of care. Working with, and believing in a true public health philosophy to midwifery care embraces a social model that places the woman and her family at the heart of her care. The underpinning theory for a social model of midwifery care is synonymous with that of woman-centred care; a fundamental concept necessary for quality midwifery services. Woman-centred care encapsulates terms such as trust, respect, empowerment, facilitation, and working in partnership with the woman and her family to maximise health outcomes. How midwives interact with women and families is fundamental to the outcome for mother and baby.

The 'medical model' of childbearing defines pregnancy as a potentially pathological process, only normal in retrospect and does not take into account all the factors outlined in the description of the 'social model' above. Care in hospital settings is central to the medical model, and according to the medical model, birth is a 'medical problem' (Wagner 1994). A 'social model' of maternity care views pregnancy and birth as normal life events. It recognises that most women are fit and well, and provides care appropriate to the individual's needs. The social model acknowledges childbearing as part of the fabric of people's lives. Care is largely community-based, linked with other agencies. Social support is recognised to be of equal importance to professional input in influencing outcomes for the woman, her baby and family. To develop a thorough understanding of how these contrasting models of care have evolved, it is helpful to consider briefly the development of midwifery as an occupation over the past 100 years or so. As Hunt vividly describes:

> . . . to be a midwife is a social and cultural experience . . . which will differ from culture to culture and over time. To be a midwife in a Bronze Age encampment, or in the court of a Stuart monarch, in the slums of 19th century Manchester and in a modern hospital are different experiences which carry different meanings
>
> (Hunt and Symonds 1995)

The social model of care and its relevance to midwifery public health

The 20th century witnessed profound and unprecedented changes in maternity care in the United Kingdom. These changes focused on two interconnected areas: the care providers, and where care was provided, and were all made with the underlying aim of reducing maternal and infant mortality and morbidity. This period also saw a dramatic improvement in outcomes for mothers and babies. In the early years of the 20th century, perinatal and maternal mortality stood at 110 and 5 per thousand respectively (Tew 1995). The improvement in morbidity and mortality rates can be clearly linked to improvements in public health and general medical advances over the course of the century. Improved housing and sanitation, the availability of contraception, the development of antibiotics and blood transfusions and improved nutrition for civilians during the Second World War all contributed to the reduction in maternal and perinatal mortality. The first governmental report to take all these factors into consideration and to examine the evidence available, concluded that:

> . . . it is no longer acceptable that the pattern of maternity care should be driven by presumption about the applicability of a medical model of care based on unproven assertions
>
> (HMSO 1992:xciv)

This statement in the Winterton Report is highly significant because it paved the way for a reshaping of maternity care to re-integrate the principles of public health into development of services and to acknowledge the impact of social factors on the outcome of pregnancy.

Institutional-centred and woman-centred care

Over the course of the 20th century, place of birth altered dramatically, with the percentage of babies born in hospital increasing steadily, from 15% in 1927 to 54% in 1946 (Peretz 1990:34), until by 1992, 97% occurred in hospital (OPCS 1994). The rationale for encouraging women to give birth in hospital was to improve maternal and perinatal mortality and morbidity. This shift in the locus of place of birth was led by a series of government recommendations and reports, culminating with the Peel Report in 1970 (HMSO 1970), which recommended that 100% of women should be encouraged to give birth in hospital. Recognising that this would inevitably mean that women's experience of care would be fragmented, it was justified on the grounds of being a more efficient service and easier to organise.

The shift from a community-based model of maternity care, with most women giving birth at home, to an institution-centred model continued inexorably, until by the 1970s and 1980s, services were provided predominantly in large, purpose-built units led by obstetric consultants. It was not until the 1990s, with the publication of the Winterton Report (HMSO 1992) and Changing Childbirth (DoH 1993) that policy on maternity care, including guidance on place of birth, was based on evidence. The Winterton Report stated clearly that it was no longer justified to encourage women to give birth in hospital on grounds of safety. The report was highly significant in terms of public health midwifery, because it led to the redevelopment of community-based maternity services that took into account the particular needs of individual women and their communities. It challenged the assumption that had grown steadily throughout the 20th century that women would go to where the caregivers were based rather than vice versa.

Ironically, the changes in the pattern of care delivery had been counterproductive and actually caused further compromise to women already disadvantaged by poverty and ill health. For example, the policy in the 1970s and 1980s of concentrating antenatal care in hospital deterred the attendance of many women 'whose socioeconomic circumstances make their need for antenatal care more likely' (Donnison 1988). This is because it failed to take into account the competing demands and pressures in women's lives – lack of money, inadequate public transport, and caring responsibilities for other children.

Reconnecting with midwifery public health roots

In retrospect, we can see the last 25 years of the 20th century, with the increasing medicalisation of childbirth and the dramatic shift from home to hospital birth, as a time when midwives lost touch with their public health roots. Government policies since the early 1990s give a unique opportunity to re-establish this connection and acknowledge that public health and midwifery are synonymous. Every midwife, whatever her job title, has a vital role in working with individuals, families and communities to use the time of opportunity that pregnancy brings to improve health and well-being.

One unique contribution that only midwives can make to public health lies in their ability to foster, support and believe in the processes of normal physiological pregnancy, childbirth and early motherhood. While this can have benefits for all women, the impact of such childbirth has been demonstrated to contribute to the initial well-being of severely disadvantaged women and to community capacity building (Misago *et al.* 2001).

The few projects that have put this philosophy into practice seem to demonstrate that the self-esteem women and their partners gain from positive childbirth experiences spreads into community action and inter-community support. Therefore, midwifery skills in supporting, encouraging and informing – but not managing – women, can contribute directly to public health in its widest context of physical, emotional, psychological and even in some cases spiritual well-being. For this reason, the possibility of physiological childbirth should be a basic fundamental right, wherever a woman receives midwifery care, and whatever the choices or needs of the majority of women coming through the service.

Empowering women, empowering communities

Chapter 2 focuses on inequalities in health outcomes, in relation to the links between poverty and social exclusion, and morbidity and mortality in defined communities. The evidence is clear that this is reality, but there is an assumption that targeted communities are 'empty vessels', and do not have recognised experiences, knowledge and skills that can be used (HDA 2004).

On the contrary, all communities have some 'assets' in addition to risks, and seeking out those assets holds the potential for change. As described above, by empowering women towards achieving a positive birth outcome, midwives are contributing to wider family and community physical and emotional health. A positive childbirth experience may be one of the most significant events of a woman's life. Belenky *et al.* (1997) describe how many women in their study experienced giving birth as a major turning point in their lives:

> My life was really, really dull. The only thing that really stands out is the birth of my children. That's the only thing that has happened to me ever. So that's about it (Ann)
>
> (Belenky *et al.* 1997 p. 35)

A mother whose positive birth experience enhanced her well-being could be invited to describe her experience at birth education sessions or workshops in her community. Or she could simply describe what the important things were for her, and her views could be used locally to influence midwifery practice. She has the potential to influence other women, or the care of women, and to increase her self-esteem further.

Another example of this is breastfeeding. If women are successful in breastfeeding their babies they may feel willing to help others by providing peer (mother-to-mother) support in their community. This is described fully in Chapter 3. The potential benefits of facilitating this process are twofold: it may further empower the mother, whatever her background, which could cascade through her family and friends, and it could assist the midwife or healthcare worker in their role. There are many ways in which women can be engaged with maternity services, and become empowered to work alongside midwives.

This community development model of care can begin with an individual relationship between mother and midwife, but does not focus solely on individualistic solutions to a woman's health needs. Rather, it takes a community approach

> . . . which includes inter-professional co-operation . . . places individual health needs in a broader socio-economic context . . . of equal importance is the role of community development (and) involving local women in health assessment . . .
>
> (Salmon and Powell 1998:110)

Community development is the process of change in neighbourhoods and communities (HDA 2004). The approach is not familiar to midwives, yet its underpinning philosophies are parallel with woman-centred care, as they are both associated with the words 'encourage', 'facilitate', 'enable' and 'trust'. The main focus of community development is bringing people together while empowering individuals, who may become community leaders as a result of their involvement (HDA 2004).

The philosophy of woman-centred care incorporates building positive relationships between midwives and mothers that empower women to take the lead in their childbirth experience if they want to. By engaging with women in this way, midwives are contributing to a local and national strategic focus to involve service users in the development, redesign and delivery of services. Department of Health directives (DoH 2000; 2003a; 2004c; 2004d) have offered an abundance of information profiles on the importance and mechanisms of service user involvement in the NHS over the past five years.

It is often as important for an organisation to engage more with communities as it is for communities to engage more with organisations

(HDA 2004:16)

Examples of good practice: involving women in maternity services

Janet lived in a Sure Start area, and was significantly depressed. She was pregnant with her first baby, and met Mary the midwife during her antenatal appointment. Mary encouraged Janet to attend an antenatal group, but Janet declined. She asked Mary if she could see her at home, and from there, a special relationship developed. Janet felt comfortable with and trusted Mary, and when she chose to breastfeed her baby, Mary provided lots of encouragement and support.

Two years later, Janet was still breastfeeding her daughter. In addition to that, through Mary, she became involved in providing voluntary support to other mothers, both in and out of the maternity unit. Janet's success in providing peer support increased her self-esteem, and from there she applied and became involved in a local research project with midwives and mothers. She has also gone on to some paid employment, an opportunity that arose from being involved in voluntary work in the National Health Service. Janet's depression disappeared without medication, and she described her thoughts on this:

'I really have to thank Mary for how I feel today. She helped me to believe in myself and successfully breastfeed. I never imagined I would be doing all the things I am doing now, and feel so happy.'

Social capital

Increasing employment or chances of employment through voluntary work and access to training contributes to building capacity in local communities and has, therefore, the potential to increase social capital. The Health Development Agency (2004) described social capital as

... the network and trust between people, which can be highly significant in building strong communities, combating social exclusion and providing a basis for long term economic development

(HDA 2004:13)

Kritsotakis and Garmarnikow (2004) explore the relationship between social capital and health, and cite the work of Robert Putnam (1995), whose work has generated interesting theories based on studies in the north and south of Italy, and the USA. Policy makers have become interested in the notion of the potential contribution of social capital in reducing health inequalities (HDA 2004), although there are others (Pearce and Smith 2003) who are more cautious and down play the notion of using social capital theory in the promotion of health, and Edmondson (2003) calls for further research in this area prior to its use in public policy.

Social capital and the midwife

When working in certain communities, midwives will see different levels of community spirit and sense of well-being:

Points for reflection

Consider an area where neighbours help each other, as part of a social network, or religious or cultural binding. Close-knit communities may include individuals who share life skills with others, and provide support to the community that promotes high spirit and well-being.

In contrast, reflect upon an area of deprivation where you work, a street that is neglected and deteriorating, or a particularly impoverished housing estate. For individuals living in them, a life of fear and uncertainty may exist due to unemployment or high crime rates, which may result in increased levels of depression or dependency on drugs and alcohol. Social support or networks are limited, which leads to isolation and disempowerment.

Literature relating to individual and community social capital and midwifery is limited, although Walsh (2006) uses the concept to demonstrate the positive effects of working in a birth centre. Walsh describes the community spirit in the workplace that infiltrates the worker's families.

By engaging with mothers as described above, and encouraging their involvement in maternity services either through consultation exercises or voluntary work, midwives have the potential to increase social capital. An example of this can be seen above, when local women were given support and training to deliver health messages to women with gestational diabetes. The women involved described how they feel part of a team working in the community and hospital with midwives and obstetricians. They feel valued and useful, and have developed new knowledge and skills. One of the most important repercussions from this is that they describe how they have taken these skills home, and shared them with members of their family and wider community.

Conclusion

> Remember the double vulnerability of childbirth, poverty and despair, and pay extra attention to the poor and dispossessed. Your work takes you to the centre of life itself. Remember that and your position in the world. Done well, your work will resonate through society and forward into future generations
>
> (Page 1996:252)

This encapsulates the impact midwives can have by embracing a public health approach to our role. This impact will be measured and – more importantly – experienced, far beyond our lifetimes.

Key implications for midwifery practice

- Think carefully about individual women's backgrounds, and examine your approach to care.
- Aim to be non-judgmental in your approach to care.
- Think about the community where you work. Are there any individual or groups of women who have different needs from the services you provide? Ask them!
- Find out where the local Children's Centres are, and ask what health services are provided there. Think about how you could care for women in those centres.

References

Acheson Report: see Department of Health (1998).

Ashton J, Seymour H (1998) *The New Public Health*. London, Open University Press.

Barker D, Clark P (1997) Fetal under-nutrition and disease in later life. *Reproduction* 2(2): 105–12.

Belenky MF, Clinchy BM, Goldberger NR, Tarule JM (1997) *Ways of Knowing: the development of self, voice and mind*. New York, Basic Books.

Black Report: see HMSO (1980).

Burden ML, Woghiren O, Burden AC (2000) Diabetes in Afro Caribbean and Indio Asian ethnic minority people. *Journal of Royal College of Physicians of London* 34(4): 343–46.

Confidential Enquiry into Maternal and Child Health (CEMACH) (2004) *Why Mothers Die* 2000–2002. London, RCOG Press.

Cumberlege Report: see Department of Health (1993).

Department for Education and Skills (2004) *Every Child Matters: Change for Children*. London, The Stationery Office. www.dfes.gov.uk/everychildmatters/ (accessed 4/12/06).

Department of Health (1993) *Changing Childbirth*: report of the Expert Maternity Group (Cumberlege Report). London, HMSO.

Department of Health (1998) *Independent Inquiry Into Inequalities In Health* (Chair: Sir Donald Acheson). London, The Stationery Office.

Department of Health (1999a) *Saving Lives: Our Healthier Nation*. London, The Stationery Office.

Department of Health (1999b) *Making a Difference: strengthening the nursing, midwifery and health visiting contribution to health and healthcare*. London, The Stationery Office.

Department of Health (2000) *The NHS Plan: a plan for investment, a plan for reform*. London, The Stationery Office.

Department of Health (2002) *Health and Neighbourhood Renewal*. London, The Stationery Office.

Department of Health (2003a) *Choice, Equity and Responsiveness*. London, The Stationery Office.

Department of Health (2003b) *Tackling Health Inequalities: a programme for action*. London, The Stationery Office.

Department of Health (2004a) *National Service Framework for Children, Young People and Maternity Services*. London, The Stationery Office.

Department of Health (2004b) *Public Service Agreement*. www.dh.gov.uk/AboutUs/HowDHWorks/ServiceStandardsAndCommitments/DHPublicServiceAgreement/fs/en (accessed 4/12/06).

Department of Health (2004c) *Building on the Best*. London, The Stationery Office.

Department of Health (2004d) *Patient and Public Involvement in Health: the evidence for policy implementation*. London, The Stationery Office.

Department of Health (2004e) *Choosing Health: Making Healthy Choices Easier*. London, The Stationery Office.

Department of Health (2006) *Our Health, Our Care, Our Say: a new direction for community services*. London, The Stationery Office. www.dh.gov.uk/PublicationsAndStatistics/Publications/PublicationsPolicyAndGuidance/fs/en (accessed 4/12/06).

Donnison J (1988) *Midwives and Medical Men*. Heinemann Historical Publications Ltd.

Edmondson R (2003) Social capital: a strategy for enhancing health? *Social Science and Medicine* 57: 1723–33.

Edwards N (2000) Women planning home births: their own views on their relationships with midwives. In Kirkham M (ed) (2000) *The Midwife–Mother Relationship*. London, Macmillan Press.

English National Board (2001) *Midwives in Action: a resource*. London, ENB.

Health Development Agency (2004) *Developing Healthier Communities*. London, HDA.

Health Development Agency (2005) *Health Needs Assessment: a practical guide*. London, HDA.

Her Majesty's Stationery Office (1970) *Domiciliary Midwifery and Maternity Bed Needs: Report of the Standing Maternity and Midwifery Sub-Committee.* (Peel Report). London, HMSO.

Her Majesty's Stationery Office (1980) *Inequalities in Health* (Black Report). London, HMSO.

Her Majesty's Stationery Office (1992) *Commons Select Committee Report on Maternity Services* (Winterton Report). London, HMSO.

Hunt S (2004) *Poverty, Pregnancy and the Healthcare Professional*. London, Books for Midwives.

Hunt S, Symonds S (1995) *The Social Meaning of Midwifery*. Basingstoke, Macmillan.

Kritsotakis G, Garmarnikow E (2004) What is social capital and how does it relate to health? *International Journal of Nursing Studies* 41: 43–50.

Leap N, Hunter B (1993) *The Midwife's Tale*. London, The Scarlet Press.

Maternity Alliance (2004) *Experiences of Maternity Services: Muslim Women's Perspectives*. London, Maternity Alliance.

Misago C, Kendall C, Freitas P *et al.* (2001) From 'culture of dehumanization of childbirth' to 'childbirth as a transformative experience': changes in five municipalities in north-east Brazil. *International Journal of Gynecology and Obstetrics* 75: S67–S72.

Neile E (1997) Control for black and ethnic minority women: a meaningless pursuit. In Kirkham MJ, Perkins ER (eds) *Reflections on Midwifery*. London, Baillière Tindall.

Office for National Statistics (2002) Deaths 2002: *Childhood infant and perinatal mortality: Live births, stillbirths and linked infant deaths by mother's age and country of birth (numbers and rates)* www.statistics.gov.uk/StatBase/xsdataset.asp?More=Y&vlnk=7984&All=Y&B2.x=35&B2.y=14 (accessed 4/12/06).

Office of Population Censuses and Surveys (OPCS) (1994) *Birth Statistics* (annual). London, HMSO.

Page L (1996) Reclaiming Midwifery. *Midwives* 109(1304): 248–53.

Pearce N, Smith GD (2003) Is social capital the key to inequalities in health? *American Journal of Public Health* 93(1): 122–29.

Peel Report: see HMSO (1970).

Peretz E (1990) A maternity service for England and Wales. In Garcia J, Kilpatrick R, Richards M (eds) *The Politics of Maternity Care: Services for Childbearing Women in the Twentieth Century*. Oxford, Oxford University Press.

Putnam RB (1995) Bowling Alone: America's declining social capital. *Journal of Democracy* 6(1): 65–78.

Royal College of Midwives (2001) Position paper No 24: *The Midwife's Role in Public Health*. London, RCM.

Salmon D, Powell J (1998) Caring for women in poverty: a critical review. *British Journal of Midwifery* 6(2): 108–11.

Sandall J (2004) Normal birth is a public health issue. *MIDIRS Midwifery Digest* (suppl) 14(1): S4–S8.

Sandall J (2005) Who, when, where and how? The implications of the National Service Framework (NSF) for the maternity care workforce In Lee B (2004) *Changing Childbirth again? Implications of the NSF. Midwives* 8(4): 164.

Tew M (1995) *Safer Childbirth? A Critical History of Maternity Care*. London, Chapman and Hall.

Wagner M (1994) *Pursuing the Birth Machine*. New South Wales, ACE Graphics.

Walsh D (2006) Birth centres, community and social capital. *MIDIRS Midwifery Digest* 16(1): 7–15.

Wanless D (2002) *Securing Our Future Health: Taking a Long-Term View*. London, HMSO.

Winterton Report: see HMSO (1992).

Chapter 2
Health and Inequality:
What Can Midwives Do?

Eileen Stringer

> Equals to be treated equally and unequals unequally in propor-
> tion to the relevant inequalities
>
> (Aristotle 384–322 BC)

What is health?

For many years, the professional training of many health workers
has been underpinned by a traditional biomedical view of health
that sees health as an absence of disease or illness, and the more
disease a person has, the further away he or she is from health
and 'normality' (Naidoo and Wills 2000). In addition, western
scientific medicine has been said to adopt a technocratic approach,
viewing the body as a machine with health equalling all parts of
that machine functioning normally (Naidoo and Wills 2000).
However, the World Health Organization (WHO) has a much
broader view:

> Health, which is a state of complete physical, mental and social
> well-being, and not merely the absence of disease or infirmity,
> is a fundamental human right and that the attainment of the
> highest possible level of health is a most important world-
> wide social goal whose realisation requires the action of many
> other social and economic sectors in addition to the health
> sector
>
> (WHO 1978)

Health in unequal proportions

Several authors argue that far from ill health being a matter of bad luck, it is socially determined, leading to the more affluent members of society living longer and enjoying better health than those in disadvantaged social groups (Department of Health (DoH) 1998; Naidoo and Wills 2000; Bostock 2003; DoH 2003).

Inequalities in health have been defined as the difference in morbidity and mortality between individuals of higher or lower socioeconomic status, to the extent that these differences are perceived to be unfair (Bostock 2003). The reasons for this inequality in health are the result of a complex, wide-ranging network of factors. A wealth of scientific evidence has traced the roots of ill health to such determinants as income, education, employment, environment and lifestyle behaviours such as smoking, drinking, diet and risk-taking (DoH 1998). People who experience disadvantage in these categories are among those most likely to suffer poorer health outcomes and an earlier death compared with the rest of the population. In addition, they are more likely to be socially excluded or marginalised, which in turn compounds the negative impact on health (Naidoo and Wills 2000).

This evidence is not new; in 1980 the Black Report (DHSS 1980), in what has come to be regarded as seminal work in health inequalities, reported that if the mortality rates of occupational class I had applied to classes IV and V during 1970–1972, 74 000 lives of people under 75 would not have been lost. Shockingly, this estimate included nearly 10 000 children (Townsend, Whitehead and Davidson 1992).

In the 25 years since this report, death rates have fallen among both men and women across all social groups, however, the difference in rates between those at the top and bottom of the social scale has widened, with death rates falling more in the higher social groups (DoH 2003). This inequality is manifested in the latest, sobering national statistics: a boy living in Manchester or a girl living in Liverpool today are expected to live 8.5 years and 7.9 years less than a boy or girl living in Kensington and Chelsea (National Statistics 2005).

What does health inequality look like?

The place or environmental circumstances a person lives in can play a large part in influencing their level of exposure to health risks, including the chances and opportunities for making healthier lifestyle choices (DoH 2003). For example, people living in disadvantaged areas are more likely to find it harder to access good shopping facilities. The food that is available is often more expensive than that sold in out-of-town supermarkets and the lack of money can then make it difficult to make what are known to be healthier choices (Naidoo and Wills 2000). Poorer people also have a higher exposure to physical hazards such as environmental pollution, traffic volume and rates of road accidents (DoH 1998) and people who rent their home tend to be both poorer and in poorer health than homeowners (Macintyre, Hunt and Sweeting 1996). Poverty and debt also have an effect on people's psychological health, with those on a low income experiencing stress, depression and social isolation (Joseph Rowntree Foundation 1999).

Those living in disadvantaged areas are less likely to access health services, a phenomena sometimes referred to as the Inverse Care Law (Hart 2000), which points to the fact that those communities most at risk of ill health often have least access to a range of effective preventive services including cancer screening programmes, health promotion and immunisation (DoH 1998). The *Tackling Health Inequalities: Status Report* (DoH 2005a) demonstrates that that the take-up of health services can be inhibited by a lack of social networks, lack of role models, lack of confidence in providers and inflexible working patterns. The consequence of this is that people in disadvantaged areas might access health services in a different way; for example, they are more likely to use emergency services than preventive ones (DoH 2005a).

A life-course approach to health inequalities argues that health in later life is affected by a complex combination of factors that can occur even before birth (Davey Smith 2001; Babb, Martin and Haezewindt 2004). The health consequences of parental circumstance can start to manifest in utero with growth retardation and subsequently, low birthweight. Two principal determinants of a baby's weight at birth are the mother's pre-pregnant weight and her own birthweight. Research into the effects of a mother's nutrition on her child's later health has shown that the small size or thinness at birth of an individual is associated with coronary heart disease, diabetes and hypertension in later life (DoH 1998; Babb, Martin and Haezewindt 2004; Spencer 2004). Smoking in pregnancy is also known to be a key determinant of low birthweight and is closely linked to socioeconomic status (Babb, Martin and Haezewindt 2004). In England and Wales in 2002, the percentage of singleton births with low birthweights was higher for babies with mothers living in the more deprived areas, and overall the incidence of low birthweight babies was highest (9%) among babies registered by the mother alone (Macintyre, Hunt and Sweeting 1996; Babb, Martin and Haezewindt 2004). Babies born to women who smoke are twice as likely to have a low birthweight than babies born to non-smokers and weigh on average 200 g less (Bull, Mulvihill and Quigley 2003). In addition, infants of mothers who smoke have almost five times the risk of sudden infant death compared with infants of mothers who do not smoke (Richardson 2001).

Although the strong relationship between socioeconomic status and smoking has been discussed in Chapter 3 it is worth reinforcing the cycle of health inequalities (Babb, Martin and Haezewindt 2004). Research shows that low-income smokers, particularly lone parents, cite smoking as a way of dealing with stress and problems, although there is little to suggest that nicotine has any true sedative action (Action on Smoking and Health (ASH) 2005). Smokers may feel that cigarettes reduce stress because if they do not smoke, they feel worse (due to nicotine withdrawal) so that smoking is necessary to regularise their mood (ASH 2005).

A major indicator of the health of the population is the infant mortality rate (deaths at age under one year per 1000 live births). Although the 20th century has seen rates drop significantly, important differences exist according to certain socioeconomic factors. In the latest national health statistics, the overall infant mortality rate was 4.9 per 1000 live births. In comparison, the rate in babies registered by the mother alone was 6.3 per 1000 live births and particularly high infant mortality rates of 8.5–8.9 per 1000 live births were seen in babies of mothers born in Pakistan, the Caribbean and parts of Africa (National Statistics 2005). These statistics demonstrate the clear association between minority ethnic groups and poor health. Members of minority ethnic groups are more likely to live in the poorest 20% of local authorities and have problems accessing services that tend to be of poorer quality and not responsive to their needs (DoH 2003).

Cultural differences between social groups and their attitudes towards health can also have an impact on outcome. For example, people in higher socioeconomic groups tend to have a stronger 'locus of control' – that is, an inner, self-belief that they can change their behaviour – and believe that they determine the course of their life (Naidoo and Wills 2000). Those in lower socioeconomic groups who may struggle with everyday life do not make long-term plans and have a fatalistic view of health, believing it to be a matter of luck (Naidoo and Wills 2000). Given such beliefs and the reality of their daily lives, it is little wonder that this group of people find it hardest to change their behaviour.

As discussed in Chapters 5 and 6 there is a strong relationship between socioeconomic status and an increase in under-18 conception rates. While some young women welcome pregnancy and find it a positive and life-enhancing experience, evidence comparing teenage mothers with women aged 20–35 years demonstrated that teenage mothers and their children are at higher risk of experiencing adverse health, educational, social and economic outcomes (DoH 1998).

There is clear evidence that breastfeeding has positive health benefits for both mother and baby in the short and long term. Breastfeeding has an important contribution to make towards meeting the national target to reduce infant mortality and health inequalities. However, women from lower socioeconomic groups have lower breastfeeding rates than those from higher socioeconomic groups, and teenage mothers are half as likely to breastfeed as older women (National Institute for Health and Clinical Excellence (NICE) 2005; DoH 2004a).

Tackling health inequalities

Past governments have focused on the effect of lifestyle and individual behaviour on health. In 1992 the *Health of the Nation* strategy looked at individual responsibility for health and set specific targets to change people's behaviour. In its White Paper: *Saving Lives: Our Healthier Nation* (DoH 1999) the government rejected the 'victim-blaming' approach and offered a 'third way' in which individuals help to make themselves healthier, supported by professionals who offer advice and information, encourage people to change and equip them with the skills and confidence to make those changes.

Improving health and reducing inequalities has become a key political aim for this government, as seen by the target to reduce inequalities in health outcomes by 10% as measured by infant mortality and life expectancy at birth by the year 2010 (Hunter and Killoran 2004). A clear policy framework has been developed to achieve this aim, with the first steps being taken in July 1997, when the newly-elected government commissioned a second independent inquiry. The task was to review the evidence and identify areas for policy development likely to reduce health inequalities. This review, chaired by Sir Donald Acheson (DoH 1998), highlighted how a more co-ordinated approach could have a profound impact on the health of the nation. It produced 39 recommendations based on scientific and expert evidence, with the aim of improving health for all, but improving the health of the poorest, fastest (DoH 1998; DoH 2003). The report recommended both 'upstream' and 'downstream' policies, that is, both preventive and secondary service provision (DoH 1998), with high priority being given to reducing inequalities in women of childbearing age, expectant mothers and young children. Some of the key recommendations argued for further efforts in the promotion of breastfeeding, nutrition during pregnancy, smoking cessation programmes for pregnant women, reduction in unwanted teenage pregnancy rates, and to provide effective early childhood support and education.

The virtual tidal wave of recent public health policy clearly reflects the global agenda for health, which focuses on a whole system approach to tackling poor health and health inequalities by interlinking of social, political and economic approaches (WHO 1986; WHO 1997). These approaches can be seen in the current *Every Child Matters: Change for Children* programme (DfES 2004) and the *National Service Framework for Children, Young People and Maternity Services* (DoH 2004a), which cut across education, social and healthcare to meet the needs of children and families through Children's Centres, with an initial emphasis on the most deprived communities.

More recently, the public health White Paper *Choosing Health* signalled the government's intention to refocus the NHS into a service that improves health as well as one that treats sickness (DoH 2004b). The intention is to help more people make healthier choices and reduce health inequalities by offering practical help that focuses on targeted support to communities with the worst health and deprivation. The vision is that health improvements and tackling health inequalities will become part of the NHS main-stream planning and will be at the core of its day-to-day business (DoH 2004b).

It is important to remember that in tackling health inequalities, understanding and addressing the social and material conditions of men's and women's lives will prevent more deaths and chronic illness than any health care intervention (DoH 1998; Walters 2004).

The government showed further commitment in the publica-tion of the out of hospital White Paper *Our Health, Our Care, Our Say* (DoH 2006b), the main aims of which are to change the way services are provided in communities and make them as flexible as possible. If this is undertaken effectively, it should reinforce the recommendations of the National Service Framework and help to make care more accessible to the most disadvantaged groups by providing high quality, locally-based services.

These policy documents are excellent tools for midwives to use when wanting to provide alternative, individualised and woman focused care. Healthcare providers are performance-managed against many of the targets in the directives, and midwives should therefore familiarise themselves with the content.

Social context of women's lives from a national and global perspective

> From a health inequality perspective, gender matters. Whether or not you are born male or female can have a profound effect on your future health
>
> (Walters 2004)

Worldwide, nearly 600 000 women between the ages of 15 and 49 die every year as a result of complications arising from pregnancy and childbirth (WHO 1999). The low social and economic status of girls and women is a fundamental determinant of maternal mortality in many countries, with social status influencing a woman's access to health services, good nutrition, employment opportunities, education and the decision-making power needed to access or pay for family planning services. Some women are denied access to care when it is needed, either because of cultural practices of seclusion or because decision-making is the responsibility of other family members (WHO 1999). The largest impact of such influences is often reflected in the vastly different rates of life expectancy across the globe – for example, in England and Wales today the average life expectancy at birth for a woman is 80.83 years. In Zambia, it is 38 years – nearly half a century less (Macintyre, Hunt and Sweeting 1996; Hewitt 2005).

To understand women's health, we need to consider how a woman's day-to-day life and multiple social roles profoundly influence her experience of illness (Lorber 1997).

Women, on average, are poorer than men and often economically dependent on others. Social isolation and poverty is much more common in women and they are more likely to experience domestic or sexual violence in childhood. It can be argued that the impact of such experiences is reflected in the type of illnesses they present with. For example, anxiety, depression and eating disorders are more common in women (DoH 2002).

The Acheson report (DoH 1998) underlined the importance of socioeconomic position as the most fundamental of the social determinants of health, stating that a person's socioeconomic position arises from their education, occupation and income. It is well recognised that children represent a major factor in earning capacity and the earning differential between men and women (Bostock 2003). Although women in recent decades have entered the labour market and achieved a greater degree of economic independence, it has come in the guise of part-time or lower-paid employment. Gender inequalities in the job market and women's role as primary caregivers within the family reinforce the idea that lower-wage-earning females, rather than higher-wage-earning men, should miss work time due to family illness (Hofmann and Hooper 2001; Bostock 2003; Walters 2004).

Childcare provision has until recently remained woefully inadequate, and this limits employment opportunities, for when women do find work that fits in with family life, they are more likely to be lower paid than men and have less control over their work environment. Many women work in the public sector, and a common characteristic in recent years is a continuing restructure and streamlining of services, with the burden of work increasing for public sector workers (Walters 2004). Even when women undertake full-time employment, they are more likely to retain the bulk of household chores (Walters 2004).

The effect of the divorce rate also has a profound effect on the health of women, as they become sole earners as well as lone parents. In many European countries the number of female-led one-parent families is increasing and this increases the risks of health and social problems associated with the downward spiral of economic disadvantage (Bostock 2003). Lorber (1997) argues that a single mother in low-wage employment, for example, is less likely to have the time, energy or educational resources to practise good nutrition, to pursue healthy leisure activities or schedule medical appointments when sick, compared to a married man who is a well-paid manager. Social factors and a good level of social support are especially important in explaining women's and men's health and these factors shape health directly, by influencing individual behaviours such as smoking, drinking, weight and physical activity (Walters 2004).

The common belief is that 'women are sicker but men die quicker' and that women are more likely to report health problems whereas men have a shorter life expectancy (Walters 2004). However, although women do currently demonstrate a longer life expectancy, studies suggest that this does not necessarily lead to a better quality of life. Other recent research confirms that gender differences in health are less clear than is often assumed and in some cases, there are few or no differences between women and men, particularly if they have a similar social status in terms of, for example, professional and economic background (DoH 1998; Walters 2004).

A degree of caution is therefore required when making statements about women's health based on evidence derived from studies that do not examine gender in its widest sense, as opposed to 'sex' as a biological differential between subjects. Gender describes those characteristics of women and men that are socially determined, that contribute to our sense of who we are, the roles we adopt, the way in which we perceive others and in which they perceive us (Lorber 1997; DoH 2002; Walters 2004).

The influence of gender becomes more complex when applied to ethnicity. Women from different cultural backgrounds have different health and nutritional practices and may have differing interpretations of medical advice. Women from minority ethnic groups, notably Pakistani and Bangladeshi groups, prefer to consult with female doctors (DoH 1998). A national survey found that South Asian women, especially Pakistani and Bangladeshi women, were less likely to have had a cervical smear in the last five years. When the non-attendees were questioned, approximately half lacked basic information about cervical screening, or did not know what the test was. Once they understood the purpose of the test and its procedures, they were found to be enthusiastic about the screening (DoH 1998). To respond to these differences, the provision of sensitive maternal and child health services is of particular importance. Cultural competency training can raise awareness in health providers to the differences among patients (Hofmann and Hooper 2001).

The biggest impact on inequalities in health will come from addressing the social and material conditions of men's and women's lives and as such requires considerable political and social engineering (DoH 1998; Walters 2004). In Thailand, the need to promote social justice was embraced when what began as a health programme was transformed into a women's empowerment programme as they searched for ways to transform health. The Thai government realised that in order to promote health, they first needed to transform women's social and economic place in society (Hewitt 2005).

Engaging vulnerable groups

If health is to a large extent created by the social environment, then that environment must be the first point of intervention in preventing problems (Walters 2004). In terms of tackling health inequalities, the 'one-size-fits-all' approach has not produced equitable health outcomes, as most local health services are able to identify geographical areas or certain groups of local people who do not receive the treatment or care that they need (DoH 2003). Interventions that are traditionally provided may be considered effective in general terms, but they may be ineffective in reducing health inequalities if they are not reaching all groups. Interventions that target health inequalities can only be considered successful when they are at least as effective for the lowest socioeconomic group as for the highest (Hunter and Killoran 2004).

One method of reaching vulnerable groups is by using existing services to raise the awareness and understanding of local communities about how to improve their own health (DoH 2005b). It is important that when doing this we take account of people's different circumstances and their constraints on choice, for example, their assertiveness skills. An empowerment approach to health promotion is key. Supporting, enabling and strengthening individuals will ensure that they have the information, confidence and skills to make informed choices and participate in planning services that meet their needs (DoH 2005b).

The new patient forums supported by the Commission for Patient and Public Involvement in Health will be a key resource in this regard. The primary care trust patient forums will provide training and support to empower local communities, and in particular excluded groups, to identify issues affecting their health, and take action to influence change on those issues (DoH 2003). Local people as well as community and voluntary organisations are an invaluable source of knowledge about how appropriate or effective provision of a local service might be (DoH 2003). Tapping into this knowledge will be crucial at the strategic planning stages in order to develop an effective local response to health inequalities.

There is an opportunity for building practical links between the communities and local services by drawing in lay health workers and providing them with training to provide basic health advice and family support (DoH 2003; DoH 2006b). Strengthening communities in this way by involving them in decision-making is viewed as a way of building social capital, as does the redesigning of local jobs to widen access to employment. Decision-making in a community may require community advocacy, that is, locally elected representatives who can represent local people's concerns and views to local policy makers and decision makers (Naidoo and Wills; DoH 2005b). This has been discussed in detail in Chapter 1.

Reducing the health inequalities gap means targeting the most vulnerable and excluded members of society. Outreach services are essential in this instance and we need to be able to identify and respond in innovative ways, taking a flexible approach to meeting individual needs. Peer approaches are particularly noted for their strengths in reaching and engaging vulnerable/difficult to reach groups (DoH 2003; DoH 2004a; DoH 2006b). For example, there is evidence that in the context of substance misuse, when the peers are ex-drug users, credibility is enhanced and the peers are seen to have 'authentic knowledge' (Millward *et al.* 2004b). Peer educators can provide positive experiences for that individual and can offer potential 'gateways' to future personal and/or career development (Millward *et al.* 2004b).

One of the strongest messages to come out of recent government policy is that reducing the gap in health inequalities will not be achieved by doing 'more of the same' and that success will only come through a radical change in the way local people are 'engaged' in improving their own health, working as active partners with a wide range of local organisations and voluntary agencies (Bostock 2003; DoH 2003).

Race is another area that requires careful consideration when trying to address health inequalities. It is important not to put all members of ethnic minorities into one disadvantaged category. Grouping of minority ethnic people, such as black or South Asian, is inappropriate, merging together people who have different cultures, religion, migration history, socioeconomic status and geographical location (DoH 1998). One way of reaching members of black and minority ethnic groups is to ensure that there is representation on appropriate decision-making and advisory bodies, and that other opportunities are taken to seek the views of these communities. Liaison with key leaders in the communities can provide a sense of cultural ownership. Services providers can utilise an understanding of the norms, history, codes and beliefs within that community to plan appropriate services (DoH 2003; Babb, Martin and Haezewindt 2004; DoH 2004a; Millward *et al.* 2004b; Syme 2004).

Maternal and neonatal outcomes are poorer for women from disadvantaged vulnerable or excluded groups, and a key strategy for improving the health of the population is to develop high quality maternity services delivered in a culturally sensitive way and focused on those with high needs (DoH 1998; DoH 1994; Wilcox 1994). Standard 11 of the *National Service Framework for Children, Young People and Maternity Services* (DoH 2004a) seeks to improve equity of access to maternity services and increase the survival rates and life chances of vulnerable women and children and those from disadvantaged backgrounds, for example, teenage mothers; women who are travellers or asylum seekers; homeless women; those in prison and the disabled. In addition, women who feel stigmatised by their condition may choose not to access conventional services, for example, those who are human immunodeficiency virus (HIV)-positive, those who misuse substances or those who are experiencing domestic violence (DoH 2004a).

Inclusiveness can be promoted by ensuring that approachable and supportive antenatal services are established. Provision of information, advice and support in convenient and accessible settings encourages and enables women to engage with maternity services early in their pregnancy and to maintain contact. Sure Start local programmes initiated this process and the philosophy will be continued with Children's Centres and extended schools, which will form one of the key components in the battle against exclusion and its consequences. Multiagency workers based or working in these centres will mean they are more visible to the community. In addition, arrangements should be in place for maternity services to link into local establishments that encounter pregnant women and ensure that access to the same high standard of care is available to all and that referral pathways are agreed and active (DoH 2004a).

Working with others: improving access

The policy framework for improving health and tackling health inequalities is established, and the emphasis now must be on effective implementation (DoH 2005a). In practice, translating policy on reducing health inequalities into practice is a complex matter. We have seen how many of the determinants of health inequalities lie outside the healthcare system, and as such, health services that react to disease only have a limited contribution to make towards health improvements overall (Naidoo and Wills 2000; Syme 2004). It is therefore vital that in order to become a true 'health' service, we need to develop joint proactive strategies with other partners to prevent disease and promote health (Naidoo and Wills 2000; Syme 2004).

Many different terms can be used to describe the different ways in which people work together and it is useful to understand the definitions of some of the more commonly used terms:

Partnership	joint action between partners implying an equal sharing of power
Multiagency	organisations that belong to the same sector, such as health or education
Interdisciplinary	joint working of people with different roles or functions within the same organisation or across sectors
Intersectoral	goes beyond any one sector and may include public, private and voluntary groups (Naidoo and Wills 2000)

A shared, intersectoral responsibility for health is a central theme in much of recent social and health policy (DoH 1998; DfES 2004; DoH 2003; DoH 2004b; DoH 2006b), and while there is a general acceptance that partnership with other agencies is necessary, it requires considerable effort.

Intersectoral working brings together organisations that may not normally see themselves as having a role in promoting health. Working together increases knowledge and understanding of each other and pools knowledge and awareness of local need. Working with others requires commitment, not just from the workers themselves, but from management – a joint strategic approach is necessary if it is to succeed. Similarly, time and resources are required to make progress, as is the ability to influence change within their own organisations (Naidoo and Wills 2000).

Wilcox (1994) identifies some of the key characteristics present in successful and unsuccessful partnerships. In a successful partnership, there is:

- Agreement that a partnership is necessary
- Respect and trust between different interests
- The leadership of a respected individual or individuals
- Commitment of key interests developed through a clear and open process
- The development of a shared vision of what might be achieved
- Time to build the partnership
- Shared mandate or agenda
- The development of compatible ways of working, and flexibility
- Good communication, perhaps aided by a facilitator
- Collaborative decision-making, with a commitment to achieving consensus
- Effective organisational management

Failed or failing partnerships might demonstrate:

- A history of conflict among key interests
- One partnership manipulates or dominates
- Lack of clear purpose
- Unrealistic goals
- Differences of philosophy and ways of working
- Lack of communication
- Unequal and unacceptable balance of power and control
- Key interests missing from the partnership
- Hidden agenda
- Financial and time commitments outweighing the potential benefits (Naidoo and Wills 2000)

The current health inequality targets will not be achieved without a serious partnership across sectors. Effective leadership and management are required to ensure effective joined up policy and organisation. Future leaders and managers will need to think and reshape their services in the context of inter-relationships, rather than as a static structure (DoH 1998; Millward *et al.* 2004a). Part of the reshaping of services has already begun with the introduction of children's trusts. These will be developed as the main vehicle for delivering children's health and well-being at a local level, and will be established by local authorities working with colleagues in the health sector and other local stakeholders. The trusts will determine the services needed to drive improvements in children's health and well-being in line with the *Every Child Matters* programme (DfES 2004), which sets expectations on children's and young people's experience and identifies five principal outcomes to which all children's services should strive. The outcomes aim to ensure that every child will:

- Be healthy
- Stay safe
- Enjoy and achieve
- Make a positive contribution
- Achieve economic well-being

A large part of this strategy is to change how and where services are delivered in order to make them more accessible. Children's centres, community schools, integrated schools and extended schools are all terms used to describe programmes that put schools at the heart of the community. They bring together a range of professionals from different agencies to provide accessible services, often beyond the school day and based on the needs of children, young people and the local community (Alaszewski and Horlick-Jones 2003). Programmes that combine a range of approaches appear to offer the best prospects for an impact on health inequalities (Hunter and Killoran 2004) and this will be reflected in the variety of services on offer from each centre. Within Children's Centres, core services will include antenatal care and parental support and advice. Midwifery services will be a key partner in these developments and it is vital that there is a successful partnership between midwifery services and local authorities if we are to succeed.

The way forward for the midwifery profession

Health inequalities are stubborn, persistent and difficult to change. As midwives we have to work towards addressing not only the short-term consequences of avoidable ill health, but also the longer-term causes, that is, the effects of health inequalities that are passed on from generation to generation (DoH 2003).

In seeking to address health inequalities on the basis of the evidence, midwives face a number of challenges. First, the evidence base for tackling health inequalities is scanty. In particular, there is limited evidence about interventions designed to improve the health of particular disadvantaged communities (Hunter and Killoran 2004), or to assess the impact that maternity services have on health inequalities. The Health Development Agency finds that there is equal challenge in implementing what has been proven to work, for in some cases, 'research exists, but is not exploited' (Hunter and Killoran 2004).

Second, where evidence does exist, translating that into effective care can be difficult. Alaszewski and Horlick-Jones (2003) ask us to consider how we deliver health messages and information about the disadvantages of risky behaviour. The authors maintain that many traditional messages have been based on the assumption that the target audience is comprised of individuals who rationally review evidence and then identify and choose the best course of action to maximise the benefit to their health, when we know this is often not the case. Individuals do, however, evaluate the trustworthiness of sources of information and its relevance to their everyday lives (DoH 2005c). With this in mind, the value of the relationship between midwives, women and their families in the antenatal period should not be underestimated in terms of health promotion. A recent survey into access to maternity services demonstrated that families want more information and see the midwife as the key route for information delivery (Work Group on Health Promotion and Community Development 2006).

Local drivers for change, such as the local delivery plans that every primary care trust produces as a way of planning how services respond to national targets, can be a good starting point for midwives who want to identify what can be done locally at a practical level. For example, most local delivery plans will refer to the public health White Paper priorities for action: reducing the number of smokers; reducing obesity and improving diet and nutrition; increasing exercise; encouraging sensible drinking; improving sexual health; and improving mental health (DoH 2004b). In terms of midwifery services, the targets are to:

- Reduce smoking during pregnancy
- Increase the uptake of breastfeeding
- Reduce under-18s pregnancy
- Improve access to sexual health services
- Improve mental health and well-being
- Reduce suicide rates (DoH 2006b)

These targets provide clear direction when reviewing and planning midwifery services. However, contributing to the reduction of health inequalities is, as seen earlier, not just about the provision of direct health care. 'Frontline' clinical midwives being involved in local partnerships might achieve a positive impact on local health – for example, Sure Start programme boards or Children's Centre steering groups. Midwives have an important role in bringing public attention to those issues which are beyond the scope of individuals to change, such as social and environmental obstacles. They can push for environmental conditions that are conducive to health (Naidoo and Wills 2000) for example, by lobbying for baby-friendly facilities in local shops. In addition, each primary care trust and local authority will have a number of tools to tackle health inequalities that would benefit from midwifery input. These tools include:

- Health needs assessment
- Health equity audit
- Health impact assessment
- Integrated care pathways
- Working groups on the delivery of key strategies, including:
    - o Teenage Pregnancy Strategy
    - o *Every Child Matters*

- *National Service Framework for Children, Young People and Maternity Services*
- Children's Centres Core Offer
- *Choosing Health: Making Healthier Choices Easier*
- Neighbourhood renewal programmes

Tools for change

Working from a wider health promotion perspective is relatively new to many mainstream health services and if we are to change how we work, we need the knowledge and skills to do it. This does not mean that we have to start from the beginning; the benefits of becoming involved in wider partnerships means that we have access to knowledge, skills and services that will help us to plan effective midwifery services. For example:

- Many PCT public health departments will have a public health intelligence officer who can provide information on the local population.
- Public health specialists can provide a wealth of advice on theories and methods for health promotion.
- Online information sources include:
  - Public Health Observatories
  - National Electronic Library for Health
  - Department of Health
  - National Statistics.

Information available includes health statistics at local, regional and national levels; health promotion models; access to evidence and in some instances, provision of toolkits that help with needs assessment, planning, community participation, monitoring and evaluation.

The Health Development Agency (HDA) was originally established in 2000 to develop the evidence base to improve health and reduce health inequalities. In 2005, its functions were transferred to the National Institute for Health and Clinical Excellence (NICE) and are a valuable resource. The HDA Impact Assessment Gateway is a website that features more than 190 completed health impact assessments and toolkits. There are newly established HDA offices throughout the various regions, with established networks that run courses on health impact assessment, health needs assessment and health equity audit. These are all-important tools that are being developed to support the *Tackling Health Inequalities* programme (DoH 2003). The HDA has also produced a Working Partnership tool, which covers monitoring and evaluation (HDA 2005).

As maternity services move into the mainly uncharted territory of reducing health inequalities in the widest sense, there may be a more prominent role for action research, which will provide us with a greater understanding of the actual process of change (DoH 2006a). Action research can be used in a number of ways to generate different types of knowledge:

- When no evidence exists to support or refute current practice, or when poor knowledge, skills and attitudes exist to carry out evidence-based practice
- When gaps have been identified in service provision, or services are underused or deemed inappropriate
- When new roles are being developed and evaluated and there is a need to work across traditionally conflicting boundaries (Hunter and Killoran 2004).

The Acheson Report stated that while there are many potentially beneficial interventions to reduce inequalities in health, many of those with the best chance of reducing future health inequalities relate to present and future mothers and children (DoH 2003). The role of the midwife in this context will be challenging, but one that we embrace and in doing so, know that the way we provide care and how we promote health in the future will be transformed.

Conclusion

There is a great deal of evidence gathered about the inequalities in health that exist in relation to socioeconomic factors, gender, culture and ethnicity. We have seen that health inequalities are not just a health service issue, and that many of the major determinants of health lie beyond the reach of the National Health Service (Hunter and Killoran 2004). However, health organisations do have an important part to play, as they are a major contributor to achieving the national target on life expectancy (DoH 2005c) and the evidence has emphasised the importance of integrating health inequalities into the mainstream of service delivery with a focus on disadvantaged areas and groups.

The government has made a commitment to reduce health inequalities, and the policy framework for achieving that has been established, with the emphasis now on effective implementation.

Midwives have a key role to play in making a positive impact on health in its widest sense.

Key implications for midwifery practice

- How are you involved in the establishment of your local Children's Centres? Has partnership working played a part in that and how could it have been improved?
- Midwifery education will need to encompass health promotion theory to provide midwives with the appropriate skills and knowledge to deliver effective, preventative approaches to health.
- Maternity services will have to respond to national and local policy drivers and local need. Joint social and health needs assessment, equity audits and health impact assessments will be required.
- Intersectoral working and joint appointments across different sectors will become the 'norm'.
- Information from monitoring the take-up of services and outcomes for disadvantaged and vulnerable groups will become an essential part of inspection and commissioning of maternity services.
- Do you know your community profile? For example, what is the average female life expectancy in your area or the type and percentage of minority ethnic groups?
- What initiatives/local policy/service provision could you become involved in that would bring about most improvement in the health of women and their families?

References

Acheson Report: see DoH (1998).

Action on Smoking and Health (2005) *Smoking and Health Inequalities.* London, ASH. www.ash.org.uk (accessed 4/12/06).

Alaszewski A, Horlick-Jones T (2003) How can doctors communicate information about risk more effectively? *British Medical Journal* 327(7417): 728–31.

Babb P, Martin J, Haezewindt P (eds) (2004) *Focus on Social Inequalities.* London, Office for National Statistics.

Black Report: see DHSS (1980).

Bostock Y (2003) *Searching for the Solution: Women, Smoking and Inequalities in Europe.* London, NHS Health Development Agency.

Bull J, Mulvihill C, Quigley R (2003) Prevention of low birth weight: Assessing the effectiveness of smoking cessation and nutritional interventions. *Health Development Agency Evidence Briefing Summary.*

Davey Smith G (2001) *Health Inequalities: Lifecourse Approaches*. Bristol, Policy Press.

Department for Education and Skills (2004) *Every Child Matters: Change for Children*. London, The Stationery Office. www.dfes.gov.uk/everychildmatters/ (accessed 4/12/06).

Department of Health and Social Security (1980) *Inequalities in Health: Report of a Research Working Group* (The Black Report). London, HMSO.

Department of Health (1998) *Independent Inquiry into Inequalities in Health* (Chair: Sir Donald Acheson). London, The Stationery Office.

Department of Health (1999) *Saving Lives: Our Healthier Nation*. London, The Stationery Office.

Department of Health (2002) *Women's Mental Health: Into the Mainstream. Strategic Development of Mental Health Care for Women*. London, The Stationery Office.

Department of Health (2003) *Tackling Health Inequalities: a Programme for Action*. London, The Stationery Office.

Department of Health (2004a) *National Service Framework for Children, Young People And Maternity Services*. London, The Stationery Office.

Department of Health (2004b) *Choosing Health: Making Healthy Choices Easier*. London, The Stationery Office.

Department of Health (2005a) *Tackling Health Inequalities: Status Report on the Programme for Action*. London, The Stationery Office.

Department of Health (2005b) *Access to Maternity Services*. Research Report COI Communications No. 269911.

Department of Health (2005c) *Delivering Choosing Health: Making Healthier Choices Easier*. Gateway Ref. 4516.

Department of Health (2006a) *Best Research for Best Health: A national health research strategy*. London, The Stationery Office.

Department of Health (2006b) *Our Health, Our Care, Our Say: a new direction for community services*. London, The Stationery Office. www.dh.gov.uk/PublicationsAndStatistics/Publications/PublicationsPolicyAndGuidance/fs/en (accessed 4/12/06).

Hart TL (2000) Commentary: three decades of the inverse care law. *British Medical Journal* 320(7226): 15–18.

Health Development Agency (2005) *HDA Impact Report 2004–2005*. London, HDA.

Hewitt P (2005) Ministerial speech by the Secretary of State for Health during UK Presidency of the EU. Tackling Health Inequalities Summit, 17 October 2005.

Hofmann M, Hooper MA (2001) *Connecticut Women's Health*. Hartford CT, Department of Public Health OCLC:48197723. www.worldcatlibraries.org/oclc/48197723&referer=brief_results (accessed 13/12/06).

Hunter D, Killoran A (2004) *Tackling Health Inequalities: turning policy into practice?* Health Development Agency.

Joseph Rowntree Foundation (1999) Social cohesion and urban inclusion for disadvantaged neighbourhoods. *Foundations.* April 1999–Ref 4109. York, York Publishing Services.

Lorber J (1997) *Gender and the Social Construction of Illness.* Thousand Oaks, CA, Sage.

Macintyre S, Hunt K, Sweeting H (1996) Gender differences in health: are things really as simple as they seem? *Social Science and Medicine* 42(4): 617–24.

Millward L, Warm D, Coomber R *et al.* (2004a) *Evidence for Effective Drug Prevention in young people: a summary of findings arising from research activity to date.* Health Development Agency, May 2004.

Millward L, Warm D, Chambers J (2004b) *An interim report of the evidence for effective drug prevention research activity and learning to date.* Health Development Agency, Sep 2004.

Naidoo J, Wills J (2000) (2nd edition) *Health Promotion: Foundations for Practice.* Edinburgh, Baillière Tindall.

National Institute for Health and Clinical Excellence (2005) *Effective Action Briefing on the Initiation and Duration of Breastfeeding: Effective Action Recommendations.* University of York, NICE.

National Statistics (2005) *Health Statistics Quarterly* Winter 2005:28. www.statistics.gov.uk (accessed 18/05/06).

Richardson K (2001) Smoking, Low Income and Health Inequalities: Thematic Discussion Document Report for Action on Smoking and Health and the Health Development Agency, May 2001.

Spencer N (2004) Accounting for the social disparity in birthweight: results from an intergenerational cohort. *Journal of Epidemiology and Community Health* 58: 418–19.

Syme SL (2004) Social determinants of health: the community as an empowered partner. *Preventing Chronic Disease* 1(1): A02.

Townsend P, Whitehead M, Davidson N (1992) *Inequalities in Health.* Harmondsworth, Penguin.

Walters V (2004) The social context of women's health, BMC Women's Health 25(4): Suppl 1:S2. www.biomedcentral.com/1472-6874/4/SI/S2 (accessed 4/12/06).

Wilcox D (1994) *The Guide to Effective Participation.* Brighton, Partnership Books. www.partnerships.org.uk/guide/Sum.html (accessed 4/12/06).

Work Group on Health Promotion and Community Development (2006) *Community Toolbox.* University of Kansas. www.ncbi.nlm.nih.gov/entrez/query.fcgi?cmd=Retrieve&db=PubMed&list_uids=10968769&dopt=Citation (accessed 13/12/06).

World Health Organization (1978) *Declaration of Alma-Ata* – The international Conference on Primary Health Care, Alma-Ata, USSR 6–12 September 1978.

World Health Organization (1986) *Ottawa Charter for Health Promotion.* Geneva, WHO.

World Health Organization (1997) 4th International Conference on *Health Promotion into the 21st Century.* Jakarta, WHO.

World Health Organization (1999) *Reduction of Maternal Mortality:* a joint WHO/UNFPA/UNICEF/World Bank statement. Geneva, WHO 1999.

Chapter 3
Smoking in Pregnancy: A Growing Public Health Problem

Grace Edwards and David King

> Pregnancy offers a particular window of opportunity; it is a
> time when a woman is particularly receptive to health advice
> for both her own and her developing baby's welfare
>
> (Owen and Bolling 1996)

Background smoking in the population

What's in a cigarette? For a start there is:

- Acetone (nail varnish remover)
- Butane (lighter fuel)
- Formaldehyde (embalming fluid)
- Nicotine (addictive drug)
- Naphthalene (mothballs)
- Cadmium (battery fluid)
- Carbon monoxide (poisonous gas)
- Radon (radioactive gas)
- Methanol (rocket fuel)
- Hydrogen cyanide (executioner's poison)
- Tar (road surfacing)
- Lead (toxic metal)
- Ammonia (cleaning agent) (Owen and Penn 2001).

Despite this there are around 13 million people in the UK who smoke, of which 28% are men and 25% are women (DoH and ONS 2003).

Tobacco is addictive. More than 50% of heroine and cocaine users and alcoholics declare that cigarettes are more difficult to give up than their other addiction because they are so widely accessible. The addictive nature of nicotine is well established, even for those who smoke little and infrequently. One of the main reasons is that nicotine is rapidly absorbed in the bloodstream and high concentrations reach the brain in seconds. Once nicotine reaches the brain, it affects the central nervous system, inducing various emotional mood changes including a sense of relaxation and consequently decreased tension and arousal, explaining why people may smoke in stressful situations (www.Quitsmoking.about.com).

When a person stops smoking, the lack of nicotine causes physiological withdrawal symptoms including restlessness, irritability, headaches, inability to concentrate, lightheadedness or dizziness (www.Quitsmoking.about.com). However, smoking does not purely revolve around a biochemical addiction to a substance. Wider determinants, which will be discussed later in the chapter, affect the uptake and maintenance of this behaviour.

There is no doubt that smoking is dangerous. Smoking has been reported to account for 20% of all UK deaths and is a primary cause of chronic obstructive lung disease, coronary heart disease and a range of cancers (Wilkinson and Abraham 2004). The biggest killer of smokers is lung cancer, which was responsible for the deaths of 21 390 men and 13 110 women in 1999, with only 5% survival rates after five years from the diagnosis date (Mathews *et al.* 2000). Now these statistics may not concern a non-smoker, but it is something that affects the whole community in terms of cost. The financial burden of treating smoking related illnesses is approximately £1.7 billion per year (Twigg *et al.* 2004).

Most smokers in England begin during adolescence, approximately 1% of students aged 11–12 years old claim to be regular smokers (one or more cigarettes per week). This figure then rises to between 7–17% for 13–14 year olds and up to 32% with 15–16 year olds being classed as regular smokers, indicating an increase in the prevalence of smoking with age (Wilkinson and Abraham 2004). A worrying trend found in national surveys conducted in England showed that the prevalence of adolescent smoking is higher among girls. Teenagers with a high personal income are also at increased risk of becoming smokers (Wilkinson and Abraham 2004).

In the UK, smoking also appears to be a predominantly white pattern of behaviour with rates among black women reported to be low, but Oakley points out that smoking is not a fixed cultural trait (Oakley *et al.* 1992). She also goes on to highlight that there is limited research on smoking and ethnicity.

The Labour government recognised the adverse effects of the smoking epidemic and published the White Paper *Smoking Kills* (DoH 1998). This outlines the need for smoking cessation services to provide support to adults, and sets national targets for a reduction in smoking prevalence, which were to:

- Raise the taxation on tobacco and combat its smuggling into the UK.
- End tobacco advertising, promotion and sponsorship.
- Increase health promotion campaigns.
- Protect non-smokers from second-hand smoke.
- Reduce child smoking rates from 13% to 9% or less by the year 2010, with a fall to 11% by the year 2005.
- Reduce adult smoking in all social classes from 28% to 24% or less by the year 2010; with a fall to 26% by the year 2005.

Following on from *Smoking Kills*, the NHS National Service Framework, published in July 2000, added further impetus to the development of smoking cessation treatment. The key elements were:

- From April 2001 nicotine replacement therapy (NRT) was to be made available on prescription.
- Most nicotine replacement therapy products were to go on general sale (this happened in May 2001).
- Smoking cessation services targeting 800 000 smokers successfully quitting at the four-week stage of their cessation programme by 2006 (West and Raw 2002).

Government's position on smoking in pregnancy

What strategies have been put into place by the government to help pregnant women stop smoking?

Pregnant women who smoke are identified as a priority group in the previously mentioned government white paper *Smoking Kills* (Penn and Owen 2002). The White Paper details the government's target to reduce the percentage of pregnant women who smoke from 23% to 15% by the year 2010, with a fall to 18% by the year 2005 (DoH 1998). Pregnancy is an ideal time for women and their partners who smoke to consider quitting, as it is a time when they may be eager for information, have access to health services, and are often keen to make changes in their lifestyle to make sure their baby is healthy (DoH 1998).

Smoking in pregnancy is not without a cost both financially and emotionally, both of which will be discussed in detail later in the chapter. However, providing help to pregnant women to give up smoking would amount to approximately one-third of what it takes to provide additional support for low birthweight babies (DoH 1998). This demonstrates the beneficial and immediate impact smoking cessation services can have on our economical resources.

To further aid smoking cessation in pregnancy and postpartum care the government also introduced the White Paper *Choosing Health: Making Healthier Choices Easier* in November 2004. This details how Sure Start centres have developed new programmes since 2005 to teach and support parents in understanding issues such as smoking that affect their infant's and children's social, emotional and physical development in childhood (DoH 2004).

Prevalence of smoking in pregnancy

Although smoking rates in pregnancy are beginning to decline, the latest large-scale survey in Britain found that around one in three pregnant women had smoked during the 12 months before conception. One in five smoked up until full term and then continued after the birth. Around a third of pregnant women managed to quit before or during pregnancy. However, within 10 weeks after the birth, one in four women who had managed to quit, relapsed (BMA 2004).

The rates of smoking in the UK are reflected in other countries. Numerous studies suggest that between one in five and one in three women in various developed countries report smoking during pregnancy (Lumley *et al.* 2004). Norway, Sweden and Canada have demonstrated declines from the late 1980s onwards (Lumley *et al.* 2004). Smoking prevalence in Australia was reported to decrease from 23% in 1998 to 19.5% in 2001 (Lumley *et al.* 2004). The Surgeon General's report on women and smoking in 2000 documented a decline in the US from 34% in 1965 to 22–23% in the late 1990s, but no changes were recorded from 1998 to 2000 (Lumley *et al.* 2004).

Cultural issues also affect smoking in pregnancy. Women who are migrants or refugees, despite major social disadvantages, are much less likely to smoke than women from similar backgrounds who are born in the UK (Lumley *et al.* 2004). This lower rate is also found in other countries. Studies in the US support lower prevalence in ethnically diverse groups by indicating that African American women and Hispanic women have lower rates of smoking in pregnancy than other women (Andreski and Breslau 1995; Wiemann *et al.* 1994).

Turning our attention back to the UK, another worry is the increasing rate of smoking among young pregnant women. Smoking is twice as common among 15–24-year-old pregnant women (42% of smokers) than in those aged 35 and over (21% of smokers) (Owen and Penn 2001). A study by Meadows and Dawson (2003) also suggested that the younger the mother, the more likely they are to smoke postnatally, have a higher rate of becoming pregnant again, have a higher rate of depression and anxiety, and have more negative feelings about parenting than positive ones (Meadows and Dawson 2003).

There is also a real need to target pregnant smokers as early as possible to reduce some of the risks of smoking in pregnancy. Tuthill *et al.* (1999) linked increased smoking prevalence in pregnant women with a higher risk of perinatal mortality. They found that the smoking prevalence was 37.8% in mothers of babies who died compared with 27.2% in mothers of survivors. They concluded that the chances of having a stillbirth or perinatal death are more than 1.5 times greater for smokers than for non-smokers (Tuthill *et al.* 1999).

Wider determinants of smoking in pregnancy

Smoking and social class

There is no doubt that there is a link between smoking and social class. It seems that the greater the level of socioeconomic deprivation, the higher the rate of smoking. In England, smoking rates are lowest in the South at around 24%, but highest in London and the North, at around 29% (White and Watt 2002).

Unfortunately, sociodemographic patterns also follow suit in pregnancy. Trends in the UK indicate that women of a young age (under 20) with a poor education, low income, low employment status (i.e. unemployed or in manual work) are more likely to continue smoking during pregnancy (BMA 2004). Other factors include marital status, parity and age (Hutchison *et al.* 1996). Dorsett and March (1998) found that a single mother on benefits and living in council accommodation, with a poor level of education has an 80% chance of being a smoker (BMA 2004). Previous experience is also likely to influence women in pregnancy. Women who have smoked during a previous pregnancy are also less likely to quit, especially if the birth went without complications and the infant is healthy (BMA 2004).

However, the main socioeconomic factor highly associated with smoking in pregnancy is poverty, with the poorest women being the likeliest to smoke (Penn and Owen 2002). Bridgewood *et al.* (2000) highlighted this relationship by demonstrating a gradient in smoking prevalence with social class. In social class I, around 15% of men and 14% of women smoke cigarettes. In social class V, smoking prevalence reaches 45% for men and 33% for women. This transcends into very high levels among the deprived groups, where smoking prevalence reaches over 70% and is about 90% in homeless people sleeping rough (Bridgewood *et al.* 2000). Linked to poverty and financial situation is, of course, employment status. Women in manual work are four times more likely to smoke during pregnancy than those in non-manual work. It has been shown that just 4% of professional women smoke, compared with 26% in lower-skilled occupations (BMA 2004).

Poverty also affects children's exposure to second-hand smoke. Jarvis and Wardle (1999) also reported that 54% of babies and young children from poorer backgrounds are exposed to passive smoking, compared with 18% of those from more affluent backgrounds (Action on Smoking and Health (ASH) 2006a). Graham (1993) further highlighted the effects of poverty on smoking in single mothers by reporting reasons such as 'I smoke more if I've got bills coming in' and 'I tend to get worried. Like Christmas is coming and I'm not able to afford things I want.'

Family and peer influences

Family and peer groups have the greatest influence on people who smoke and midwives should appreciate this. The biggest influences appear to be having a partner who smokes, friends of the opposite sex, having a sibling who is a smoker and the social influences of parents and peers (O'Callaghan *et al.* 1999; Penn and Owen 2002). Influence of peer groups has also been cited on numerous occasions as a major cause for the adoption of smoking in adolescents. Another train of thought suggests that peer pressure may be an uncertain factor for causing smoking behaviour. It may be that young people simply associate with adolescents of similar backgrounds and interests who smoke (Eiser *et al.* 1989).

In pregnancy there appears to be a link between social class and smoking rates of partners. Pregnant women whose partners worked in manual employment were more likely to smoke than those with partners in non-manual work (Penn and Owen 2002).

Another interesting finding is that even though parents themselves may smoke, they more than often disapprove of their children smoking (Eiser *et al.* 1989) and parental opposition is often stronger for girls than boys, but there is still a major public health issue for children who are exposed to second-hand smoke.

Passive smoking

In the UK, 42% of British children live in a household where at least one person smokes (ASH 2006a). Passive smoking has been well documented as a cause of bronchitis, pneumonia, and coughing, wheezing, asthma attacks, middle ear infection and possibly cardiovascular and neurobiological impairment in children (ASH 2006b).

Studies have also associated exposure to second-hand smoke with sudden infant death syndrome (Letson *et al.* 2002). A confidential enquiry into stillbirths in the UK concluded that in households where only the father smoked the risk of cot death increased 2.5 times (Royal College of Obstetricians and Gynaecologists (RCOG) 1996).

The United Kingdom has approximately one in five pregnant non-smokers who cohabit with another person who smokes and who are therefore exposed to second-hand smoke during pregnancy (BMA 2004). It is estimated that second-hand smoke causes more than 17 000 children each year to be admitted to hospitals in the UK with respiratory illnesses. The cost of this care has been approximated at £167 million, based on prices as of 1997 (BMA 2004).

Passive smoking still also remains a public health issue in pregnancy, even though research has revealed a strong public opinion that pregnant women should be protected against it, as should children and people with asthma and heart disease (Christakopoulou and Dawson 2004). A review of the evidence conducted in the US by the Surgeon General's office concluded that on average, infants born to women exposed to second-hand smoke during pregnancy are 40–50 g lighter than those born to women who are not exposed (BMA 2004). This may not seem to be very important at birth, but there is an increasing body of knowledge that suggests that being born small has an effect on your health for the rest of your life, Barker *et al.* in 1992 first put forward the theory that babies who had intrauterine growth retardation were at increased risk of early mortality in adulthood from obesity, diabetes and coronary heart disease. This influence will be discussed later in the chapter.

Second-hand smoke in the workplace can also affect pregnancy, even when this exposure is relatively low. In pregnant non-smokers exposed to second-hand smoke, it is estimated that the risk of having a low-birthweight baby is increased by 20% (BMA 2004).

Pregnant women who are exposed to other people's cigarette smoke might also be raising their baby's risk of developing cancer in childhood (Sorohan *et al.* 1997a). Many countries, including the UK, have now agreed to ban smoking in the workplace and in pubs and clubs to protect workers from second-hand smoke.

Effects of smoking on reproduction and child health

Smoking in pregnancy has the potential to impact heavily on sexual, reproductive and child health. It can have a far reaching effect on the outcome of pregnancy, including:

- An increase in the rate of spontaneous abortions
- Stillbirth
- Premature rupture of the membranes
- Premature placental detachment
- Adverse effect on fetal brain development
- Preterm births
- Low birthweight infants
- Birth defects
- Neonatal death
- Sudden infant death syndrome (SID) (BMA 2004; Blair *et al.* 1996a, b; Hutchison *et al.* 1996; Golding 1994a).

To understand how smoking adversely affects pregnancy, it is useful to understand a little bit about the physiological effects of smoking. Nicotine and carbon monoxide, which is a by-product of cigarette smoke, decreases the availability of oxygen to the fetus (Hutchison *et al.* 1996; Benowitz and Dempsey 2004).

Haemoglobin binds and transports oxygen in blood vessels throughout the body and passes over the placental barrier to provide oxygen for the fetus. Carbon monoxide binds with 200 times more affinity to maternal and fetal haemoglobin, displacing oxygen and also impairing its release to the fetus resulting in cellular hypoxia. This may result in fetal growth retardation and low birthweight. Chronic carbon monoxide exposure and nicotine exposure have also been shown to have detrimental effects on fetal brain development in animal studies (Benowitz and Dempsey 2004).

Nicotine is known to cause vasoconstriction, which may restrict placental blood flow and reduce the supply of the nutrients and oxygen to the fetus (Benowitz and Dempsey 2004). More documented risks surrounding fetal exposure to nicotine focus on the increased risk of sudden infant death syndrome. It is believed that sudden infant death syndrome results from an abnormality in the cardiovascular/respiratory response to hypoxia (Benowitz and Dempsey 2004). Large-scale research in the UK has shown a direct link between sudden infant death syndrome and smoking (Blair *et al.* 1996a, b).

Nicotine levels are also present in the amniotic fluid, and because the fetus swallows amniotic fluid continually there may be a risk of ongoing exposure (Benowitz and Dempsey 2004). Nicotine is broken down in the body into cotinine. A build up of cotinine can cause uterine contractions, possibly resulting in the onset of premature labour (Dahlström *et al.* 2004). Nicotine has also been shown to affect fetal heartrate (Benowitz and Dempsey 2004).

Reproductive health risks are commonly reported in smoking and pregnancy, one of the main problems of which is an increased incidence of ectopic pregnancy among smokers (Sariaya *et al.* 1998). This may be because cigarette smoke suppresses the normal rhythmic movement of the cilia, and slows down the passage of the embryo along the fallopian tube (Sariaya *et al.* 1998). Typically studies have found that in women who smoke, the risk of ectopic pregnancy is increased by 1.5–2.5 times (BMA 2004).

Smoking may also affect fertility in both men and women. Baird *et al.* (1999) reported smokers were 3.4 times more likely than non-smokers to have taken more than a year to conceive. Other research suggests that fertility of smokers is 72% that of non-smokers (Baird *et al.* 1999). However, there is also evidence that if women give up smoking before conception, their fertility returns to the level of a person who never smoked (US Public Health Service 1980).

Smoking has also been linked to male impotence, with a large study in the US indicating that twice as many men who smoked suffered erectile dysfunction compared with non-smokers (Tengs and Osgood 2001).

There are some indications from the Avon Longitudinal Study of Pregnancy and Childhood that smokers' children's reproductive health is also affected (Golding 1994b). Daughters of mothers who smoked in pregnancy may have an earlier menarche and once pregnant, have an increased risk of bleeding and miscarriage in the first trimester. Sons of mothers who smoked during pregnancy have an increased likelihood of undescended testes (Golding 1994b).

There is also a great deal of evidence to link respiratory disease in infants with cigarette smoking (Cunningham *et al.* 1994; DiFranza and Lew 1996; Spitzer *et al.* 1998; Tager *et al.* 1995). These children are likely to have decreased lung function, with resultant respiratory problems and increased ear infections. There is also suggestive evidence that parental smoking may increase the risk of some childhood cancers (Sorohan *et al.* 1997a, b) and also have an effect on cognitive function and behaviour in adolescence (Sexton *et al.* 1994).

If adolescents smoke this can lead to asthma, shortness of breath, allergic symptoms, respiratory tract infections and high blood pressure. However, as the smoker matures into adulthood the effects on lifespan become more apparent (Wilkinson and Abraham 2004). A 35-year-old woman who smokes cigarettes can expect to die on average six years earlier than a woman who has never smoked. One in seven women aged 35 who continue to smoke cigarettes can expect to die before the age of 65; her life span will be curtailed by 5.5 years. Overall, approximately one in every two smokers (51% of males and 45% of females) will die prematurely as a result of smoking (Mathews *et al.* 2000).

Smoking and breastfeeding

It is suggested that women who smoke during pregnancy are less likely to breastfeed and more likely to wean their infants earlier (Saunders 1996). A study conducted in Australia found that 91% of breastfeeding initiation was recorded for non-smokers, 89% for women smoking between 1–9 cigarettes, 83% for 10–20 cigarettes, and 78% for 21 or more cigarettes (Amir and Donath 2002).

Various reasons have been provided to explain the occurrence of a drop in breastfeeding rates in smokers. Nicotine has been discovered to be present in the mother's breastmilk, where levels are reported to be three times higher than the level in the mother's plasma. Knowledge of which can be off-putting to smokers wishing to breastfeed (Amir and Donath 2002).

Physiologically, nicotine is believed to suppress prolactin, the hormone responsible for lactation (Amir and Donath 2002). Nicotine's ability to constrict blood vessels is also a previously reported side effect of smoking. It is also believed that by decreasing the blood flow to the breast tissue nicotine suppresses oxytocin, another hormone responsible for the mother's milk ejection response (Donath *et al.* 2004).

Oxytocin and prolactin are released when the mother's nerve endings in the nipple are stimulated. These nerve endings are connected to the hypothalamus section of the brain. Once stimulated, prolactin is released from the anterior pituitary section of the hypothalamus and oxytocin from the posterior pituitary (Amir 2001). However, it has not been shown that nicotine has a consistent negative physiological effect on lactation. Nafstad *et al.* (1996) reported that 41% of Norwegian women who smoked were still breastfeeding at six months postpartum. Therefore it is likely that psychological and sociological factors also contribute to lower rates of breastfeeding among smokers (Amir and Donath 2002).

Breastmilk production is strongly associated with mental attitude towards breastfeeding, it is said to be a 'confidence trick'. For example, Feher *et al.* (1989) noted mothers using a relaxation cassette expressed a 63% rise in breastfeeding initiation than a control group with no intervention (Amir and Donath 2002). It has also been documented that some women perceive themselves to be poor producers of milk. This is a common reason for stopping breastfeeding when it is not necessarily the case (Amir 2001).

Social factors are also believed to play a major part; in most developed countries there are similarities between those women who smoke and those who artificially feed their infants (Amir 2001). They tend to be younger, less educated and have lower incomes than non-smokers and those women who breastfeed. Non-smoking mothers who are cohabiting with a partner who smokes have also been identified as more likely to give up breastfeeding (Amir 2001). As the amount of cigarettes smoked by a woman's partner increased, the woman became more negative about breastfeeding (Amir 2001).

Whatever the cause – psychological or physiological – women who are postpartum and smoke should be encouraged to breastfeed. The health risks of artificial feeding and smoking far outweigh those of smoking and breastfeeding as the infant is not receiving the immunoprotective properties of the breastmilk that aid development of the immune system (Amir 2001).

Why people stop and why people do not

Despite the vast amount of literature and research that exists to say that smoking during pregnancy can be harmful to one's unborn child, many women still continue to do so (Hutchison *et al.* 1996). There are many reasons why women in the care of a midwife have not been able to heed their advice and stop smoking.

- They may simply want to continue smoking.
- They may have smoked throughout previous pregnancies and delivered 'healthy babies' and now possess altered health beliefs.
- They may be dependent on cigarettes for whatever reason, i.e. physical addiction, emotional or social dependency, and simply feel that their 'need to smoke' is stronger than the health arguments to give up.
- It may be that the midwife has not assessed a woman's readiness to quit accurately enough (Lancaster and Stead 2005).
- They may feel smoking cessation will result in weight gain (Bursey and Craig 2000).
- They may smoke to 'relieve anger rather than lashing out' and to 'calm down in stressful situations' (Gillies *et al.* 1989).
- Women can also rationalise that it is easier to deliver a small baby, so birthweight is not an issue likely to persuade them to give up smoking (Graham 2001).

To help explain why people attempt to stop smoking, Janz and Becker (1984) created the health beliefs model. It proposes that people weigh up the costs and benefits of the advice provided. From this, a person can judge the likelihood of a behaviour causing damaging effects (Janz and Becker 1984). The health beliefs model also postulates that for a behavioural change to take place, an individual:

- Must have an incentive to change
- Must feel threatened by their current form of behaviour
- Must feel a change would be beneficial in some way and have few adverse consequences
- Must feel competent to carry out the change (Janz and Becker 1984).

However, Prochaska and DiClemente (1986) adopted a different approach to explain behavioural change and aid midwives to tailor interventions, by devising the Transtheoretical model, which defines a 5-stage cycle through which a smoker will either progress or remain stationary:

Precontemplation	This is when a smoker is either not interested in stopping smoking, or maybe hasn't ever given it any serious thought.
Contemplation	The smoker has begun to consider giving up smoking and maybe needs some help, advice, encouragement and information to consolidate their thoughts into plans.

Preparation	They have now decided how and when they are going to stop smoking. Here the midwife can help by discussing working towards the quit date, setting the date and planning how the pregnant smoker is going to get the maximum support.
Action	The smoker is now trying to stop smoking. She is not a non-smoker at this stage but a very vulnerable recent ex-smoker, who will be tempted to have a cigarette in certain situations. The midwife can help by identifying with the woman what those difficult situations are likely to be and what she can do to avoid them.
Maintenance	The smoker has maintained cessation, they are now a non-smoker, but will still need the midwife's and health visitor's help and support (Owen and Bolling 1996).

It takes time to acquire a new behaviour, new skills, and a new sense of yourself as a non-smoker, and relapse is a normal part of the process in quitting. If the advice and support a midwife offers does not coincide with the stage a pregnant smoker is at in the transtheoretical model, it may have little or no effect (Owen and Bolling 1996).

Movement through this cycle is also not one-way traffic. People can find themselves at various points, whether this be making progress towards the maintenance stage or falling back to precontemplation (De Vries and Backbier 1994). It is hoped that by increasing the behavioural understanding of the reasons for and against smoking, the development of more effective interventions can be enabled (Johnston *et al.* 2004).

Smoking cessation interventions

Various types of smoking cessation intervention exist to aid the pregnant smoker.

Nicotine replacement therapy

Nicotine replacement therapy (NRT) is the only smoking cessation pharmacotherapy intervention used in pregnancy. Other pharmacotherapy is not recommended for use in pregnancy (Benowitz and Dempsey 2004).

As of March 2003 all NRT products were made available to pregnant women following a risk:benefit ratio assessment due to concerns over prolonged fetal exposure to nicotine (Benowitz and Dempsey 2004). This involves regular consultations and ascertaining information about a woman's smoking pattern, previous quit attempts and relapses, so that a clinical decision can be made about risk versus benefit of her using NRT (BMA 2004).

NRT is available as transdermal patches, chewing gum, nasal spray, lozenges and inhalers (Benowitz and Dempsey 2004). The most rapid dose of nicotine delivery via NRT is seen with nicotine nasal spray; followed by nicotine gum, then the inhaler, and then the lozenges. The transdermal patch releases nicotine quite slowly over a long period (Benowitz and Dempsey 2004).

Psychological support

Cessation programmes designed for pregnant women usually take a different approach by using alternative remedies (BMA 2004), and include:

- Self-help materials (e.g. anti-smoking pamphlets and videos)
- Brief intervention (e.g. advice from a midwife)
- Intensive counselling delivered to an individual or group
- Motivational interviewing
- Hypnotherapy (Lancaster and Stead 2005).

Brief intervention

The least intensive technique used is brief intervention, which can simply consist of a 10-minute chat about smoking by the smoking cessation supporter (Aveyard *et al.* 2004). This method follows the five As model:

Ask   Identify tobacco use at the first antenatal appointment.

Advise   Advise pregnant smokers to quit by using a clear and personalised approach.

Assess   Assess a pregnant smoker's willingness to become a non-smoker. If they are willing to make an attempt, they need support.

Assist   Provide counselling and, if necessary, pharmacotherapy. Ideally the smoker should set a quit date.

Arrange   Arrange a follow-up appointment to assess progress, preferably within the first week after the quit date (www.respiratoryreviews.com).

Counselling

More intensive interventions are seen with counselling, which can be provided in a group setting or on a one-to-one basis. One effective format of individual counselling is known as motivational interviewing. This technique is tailored to the various stages of behavioural change depicted in the Transtheoretical model (Thyrian *et al.* 2006).

Here the midwife addresses different aspects of non-smoking, smoking, and changing smoking behaviour, depending on which stage of the model the woman is at (e.g. precontemplation or preparation) (Thyrian *et al.* 2006). The techniques utilised in motivational interviewing include:

Expressing empathy   The midwife uses reflective listening and open questions to express their understanding of each woman's situation with regards to smoking. To illustrate, the smoker may say they do so to alleviate stress and relax. Here the midwife would reflect that life is stressful and urge the woman to relax using other means.

Developing discrepancy   The woman is asked to distinguish between current behaviour and important goals by identifying the pros and cons of not smoking. In so doing she can express opposing attitudes about the stresses of caring for her child's health versus smoking to relax. It is vital that the woman does most of the talking, putting her arguments forward.

Rolling with resistance   When a woman reacts by defending her decision to smoke, the midwife must shift the approach away from this resistance. For example a woman's reaction may be 'I took up smoking again after my first baby because he was healthy.' Here the midwife must not confront this argument with documented evidence of the health risks. A better response would be 'What are your thoughts on smoking after the birth?'

Supporting self-efficacy   The midwife should take any given opportunity to enhance a woman's confidence in her ability to change or maintain change. This can be achieved by discussing a woman's successful ability to abstain from smoking or congratulating them on reducing their consumption, thereby reinforcing that they have the ability to change (Thyrian *et al.* 2006).

Group counselling

Group counselling sessions are also used in smoking cessation. Two rationales have been provided for this. First they incorporate both characteristics of self-help material and intensive individual counselling techniques with lower costs per smoker. There may also be a beneficial therapeutic effect from smokers sharing their experiences and problems with others attempting to quit (Lancaster and Stead 2005).

Hypnotherapy

Another widely promoted intervention for smoking cessation is hypnotherapy. Different approaches of this technique are used; some strengthen the woman's will to stop while others weaken her desire to smoke (Abbot *et al.* 1998). The ability to focus on a treatment programme by increasing the woman's concentration is another technique used. Hypnotherapy can also incorporate training in self-hypnosis for the woman (Abbot *et al.* 1998).

Whatever the intervention used, midwives are the perfect health professionals to deliver them in practice, because they interview the mother in the early stages of pregnancy, and often maintain contact into the postnatal period (Hajek *et al.* 2001).

The midwife's role in smoking cessation

In December 1998 the Health Education Authority published smoking cessation guidelines for health professionals. The strategies they set are as follows:

- Advice on quitting should be given to smokers opportunistically during consultations.
- Specialist smokers' services should provide behavioural support on a group or individual level.
- Specialist cessation counsellors providing behavioural support should be made available to hospital patients and pregnant smokers wanting help quitting.
- Pregnant smokers should receive clear, easy-to-understand and accurate information on the risks of smoking to the fetus and be offered special support in quitting.
- Clinicians and midwives involved in discussing smoking with women or their family should receive training so that they do this effectively.
- All health professionals involved in cessation should instruct and assist smokers in the proper use of NRT (West *et al.* 2000).

Midwives are in a unique position, with the most, and probably the closest contact, with a woman during her pregnancy. Under the proposal *More Midwives More Choice* highlighted by the secretary of state in 2001, a midwife will see a woman through her entire pregnancy, and therefore has the privilege and responsibility for ensuring the mother and baby's optimum health (Owen and Bolling 1996). Their role in smoking cessation is a key one.

Pregnancy offers a particular window of opportunity; it is a time when a woman is particularly receptive to health advice for both her own and her developing baby's welfare. This offers an ideal opportunity for midwives to raise the issue (especially at the first antenatal appointment) of smoking cessation and respond with advice and help (Owen and Bolling 1996). Providing midwives with smoking cessation training produces an understanding of a pregnant woman's smoking behaviour, encourages staff to raise the issue of smoking cessation and increases confidence in delivering appropriate interventions (Bishop *et al.* 1998).

Most pregnant women know about the risks of smoking to themselves and their developing baby. They will very probably feel guilty about smoking, and expect the midwife to be disapproving. This can lead to non-disclosure of smoking, under-reporting, indifference or defiance of support (Clasper and White 1995). If a midwife strives to communicate in a facilitative and open manner, and is empathetic and takes a non-judgmental approach, she will encourage the woman to feel less threatened, more able to talk openly about her smoking and more inclined to change her habit (Clasper and White 1995).

Key implications for midwifery practice

- Be non-judgmental about other women.
- Be mindful of the complexities of some women's lives.
- Review recent government policy such as *Saving Lives: Our Healthier Nation, Smoking and Reproductive Life* and *Smoking Kills*.
- Do you know the rates of smoking in pregnancy in your area? Does it differ from neighbouring areas?
- Find out more about brief interventions and incorporate them into your practice.
- Link into your local health promotion team to find out how you can work in partnership to reduce smoking rates in pregnancy.
- Pregnant smokers should receive clear, easy-to-understand and accurate information on the risks of smoking to the fetus and be offered special support in quitting.
- Clinicians should be familiar with the cycle of behavioural change so that support may be targeted at the most appropriate time.

References

Abbot NC, Stead LF, White AR, Barnes J (1998) Hypnotherapy for smoking cessation. *The Cochrane Database of Systematic Reviews* Issue 2.

Action on Smoking and Health (2006a) *Fact Sheet No. 1. Smoking Statistics: Who Smokes and How Much.* www.ash.org.uk.

Action on Smoking and Health (2006b) *Passive Smoking Fact Sheet: The Impact on Children.* www.ash.org.uk/html/passive/html/kidsbrief.html (accessed: 4/12/2006).

Amir LH (2001) Maternal smoking and reduced duration of breastfeeding: A review of possible mechanisms. *Early Human Development* 64: 45–67.

Amir LH, Donath SM (2002) Does maternal smoking have a negative physiological effect on breastfeeding? The epidemiological evidence. *Birth* 29(2): 112–23.

Andreski P, Breslau N (1995) Maternal smoking among blacks and whites. *Social Science and Medicine* 41(2): 227–33.

Aveyard P, Lawrence T, Croghan E *et al.* (2004) Is advice to stop smoking from a midwife stressful for pregnant women who smoke? Data from a randomised controlled trial. *Preventive Medicine* 40(5): 575–82.

Baird DD, Wilcox AJ, Kramer MS (1999) Why might infertile couples have problem pregnancies? (letter comment). *Lancet* 353(9166): 1724–25.

Barker DJP (ed) (1992) *Fetal and Infant Origins of Adult Disease.* London, BMJ Publishing.

Benowitz NL, Dempsey DA (2004) Pharmacotherapy for smoking cessation during pregnancy. *Nicotine and Tobacco Research* 6 (Supp 2): S189–S202.

Bishop S, Panjari M, Astbury J, Bell R (1998) A survey of antenatal clinic staff: some perceived barriers to the promotion of smoking cessation in pregnancy. *Journal of Australian College of Midwives* 11: 14–28.

Blair PS, Fleming PJ, Bensley D *et al.* (1996a) Smoking and SIDS: results for a 1993 5-case control study for Confidential Inquiry into Stillbirths and Deaths in Infancy. *British Medical Journal* 313(7051): 191–95.

Blair P, Fleming PJ, Bensley D *et al.* (1996b) Smoking and the sudden infant death syndrome: results from 1993 5-case-control study for Confidential Inquiry into Stillbirths and Deaths in Infancy. *British Medical Journal* 313(7051): 195–98.

Bridgewood A, Lilly R, Thomas M *et al.* (2000) *Living in Britain:* Results from the 1998 General Household Survey. Office of National Statistics. London, The Stationery Office.

British Medical Association (2004) *Smoking and Reproductive Life, The Impact of Smoking on Sexual Reproductive and Child Health.* London, Board of Science and Education and Tobacco Control Resource Centre.

Bursey M, Craig D (2000) Attitudes, subjective norm, perceived behavioural control and intentions related to adult smoking cessation after coronary artery bypass graft surgery. *Public Health Nursing* 17(6): 460–67.

Christakopoulou S, Dawson J (2004) *Survey of Residents' Attitudes to Second-Hand Smoke in Liverpool.* Liverpool, SmokeFree Liverpool Organisation.

Clasper P, White M (1995) Smoking cessation interventions in pregnancy: practice and views of midwives, GPs and obstetricians. *Health Education Journal* 54: 150–62.

Cunningham J, Dockery D, Speizer F (1994) Maternal smoking during pregnancy as a predictor of lung function in children. *American Journal of Epidemiology* 139(12): 1139–52.

Dahlström A, Ebersjö C, Lundell B (2004) Nicotine exposure in breastfed infants. *Acta Paediatrica* 93(6): 810–16.

Department of Health (1998) *Smoking Kills: A White Paper on Tobacco.* London, The Stationery Office.

Department of Health and Office for National Statistics (2003) *Statistics on Smoking: England, 2003.* London, Office for National Statistics.

Department of Health (2004) *Choosing Health: Making Healthy Choices Easier.* London, The Stationery Office.

De Vries H, Backbier E (1994) Self-efficacy as an important determinant of quitting among pregnant women who smoke: the phi-pattern. *Preventive Medicine* 23(2): 167–74.

DiFranza JR, Lew RA (1996) Morbidity and mortality associated with the use of tobacco products by other people. *Paediatrics* 97(4): 560–68.

Donath SM, Amir LH, ALSPAC Study Team (2004) The relationship between maternal smoking and breastfeeding duration after adjustment for maternal infant feeding intention. *Acta Paediatrica* 93: 1514–18.

Dorsett R & March A (1998) *The Health Trap: Poverty, Smoking and Lone Parenthood*. London, PSI.

Eiser R, Morgan M, Gammage P, Gray E (1989) Adolescent smoking: Attitudes, norms and parental influence. *British Journal of Social Psychology* 28: 193–202.

Feher SDK, Berger LR, Johnson JD and Wilde JB (1989) Increasing Breast Milk Production for Premature Infants With a Relaxation/Imagery Audiotape. *Pediatrics* 83(1): 57–60.

Gillies P, Madeley RJ, Power FL (1989) Why do pregnant women smoke? *Community Medicine* 103: 337–43.

Golding J (1994a) Reproductive risks for babies of pregnant smokers. *Healthlines* March: 3.

Golding J (1994b) The consequences of smoking in pregnancy. *Newsletter for Professionals, ALSPAC* (Avon Longitudinal Study of Pregnancy and Childhood).

Graham H (1993) When life's a drag: women, smoking and disadvantage. London, HMSO.

Graham H (2001) Smoking in pregnancy: the attitudes of expectant mothers. *Social Science and Medicine* 10: 399–405.

Hajek P, West R, Lee A *et al.* (2001) Randomised controlled trial of a midwife-delivered brief smoking cessation intervention in pregnancy. *Addiction* 96: 485–94. www.respiratoryreviews.com/oct00/rr_oct00_tobacco.html (accessed 4/12/06).

Hutchison KE, Stevens VM, Collins FL (1996) Cigarette smoking and the intention to quit among pregnant smokers. *Journal of Behavioural Medicine* 19(3): 307–316.

Janz NK, Becker MH (1984) The Health Belief Model: a decade later. *Health Education Quarterly* 11(1): 1–47.

Jarvis M, Wardle J (1999) Social patterning of individual health behaviours: the case of cigarette smoking. In Marmot M, Wilkinson R (eds) *Social Determinants of Health*. Oxford, Oxford University Press.

Johnston DW, Johnston M, Pollard B *et al.* (2004) Motivation is not enough: prediction of risk behaviour following diagnosis of coronary heart disease from the theory of planned behaviour. *Health Psychology* 23(5): 533–38.

Lancaster T, Stead LF (2005) Individual behavioural counselling for smoking cessation. *The Cochrane Database of Systematic Reviews* 2. Chichester, John Wiley.

Letson GW, Rosenburg KD, Wu L (2002) Association between smoking during pregnancy and breastfeeding at about 2 weeks of age. *Journal of Human Lactation* 18 (4): 368–71.

Lumley J, Oliver SS, Chamberlain C, Oakley L (2004) Interventions for promoting smoking cessation during pregnancy. *The Cochrane Database of Systematic Reviews* 4. Chichester, John Wiley.

Mathews F, Yudkin P, Smith RF, Neil A (2000) Nutrient intakes during pregnancy: the influence of smoking status and age. *Journal of Epidemiology and Community Health* 54: 17–23.

Meadows S, Dawson N (2003) Teenage mothers and their children: Factors affecting their health and development. (Part of the contribution to the Social Exclusion Unit publication on Teenage Pregnancy). www.dh.gov.uk/PolicyAndGuidance/ResearchAndDevelopment/ ResearchAndDevelopmentAZ/MotherAndChildHealth/ MotherAndChildHealthArticle/fs/en?CONTENT_ID=4016317&chk= ERCV5W (accessed 13/12/06).

Nafstad P, Jaakkola JJ, Hagen JA *et al.* (1996) Breastfeeding, maternal smoking and lower respiratory tract infections. *European Respiratory Journal* 9: 2623–29.

Oakley A, Brannen J, Dodd, K (1992) Young people, gender and smoking in the United Kingdom. *Health Promotion International* 7(2): 75–88.

O'Callaghan FV, Callan VJ, Baglioni A (1999) Cigarette use by adolescents: attitude-behaviour relationships. *Substance Use and Misuse* 34(3): 455–68.

Owen L, Bolling K (1996) Smoking in pregnancy: developing a communications strategy for smoking cessation (Unpublished work).

Owen LA, Penn GL (2001) Smoking and Pregnancy: *A Survey of Knowledge, Attitudes and Behaviour 1992–1999*. London, Health Education Authority.

Penn G, Owen L (2002) Factors associated with continued smoking during pregnancy: analysis of sociodemographic, pregnancy and smoking-related factors. *Drug and Alcohol Review* 21(1): 17–25.

Prochaska JO, DiClemente CC (1986) Toward a comprehensive model of change. In Miller, WR, Heather N (eds) *Treating Addictive Behaviours: Processes of Change*. New York, Plenum Press: 3–27.

Quit smoking website: www.Quitsmoking.about.com (accessed 4/12/ 2006).

Royal College of Obstetricians and Gynaecologists (1996) *Confidential Enquiry into Stillbirths and Deaths in Infancy*, 5th Report. London, RCOG.

Sariaya M, Berg CJ, Kendrick JS *et al.* (1998) Cigarette smoking as a risk factor for ectopic pregnancy. *American Journal of Obstetrics and Gynaecology* 178: 493–98.

Saunders S (1996) Smoking and breastfeeding. *Child Antenatal Nutrition Bulletin* 11: 2–3.

Sexton M, Fox NL, Hebel JR (1994) Prenatal exposure to tobacco II: Effects on cognitive functioning at age 3. *Journal of the American Medical Association* 251: 911–15.

Sorohan T, Lancashire RJ, Hulten MA, Peck I, Stewart AM (1997a) Childhood cancer and parental use of tobacco: Deaths from 1953 to 1955. *British Journal of Cancer* 75(1): 134–38.

Sorohan T, Prior P, Lancashire RJ *et al.* (1997b) Childhood cancer and parental use of tobacco: Deaths from 1971 to 1976. *British Journal of Cancer* 76(11): 1525–31.

Spitzer WO, Lawrence V, Dales R *et al.* (1998) Links between passive smoking and disease: A best evidence synthesis. A report of the working group on passive smoking meta analysis. *Clinical and Investigative Medicine* 13(1): 17–42.

Tager I, Ngo LJ, Hajrahan J (1995) Maternal smoking during pregnancy: effects on lung function during the first 18 months of life. *American Journal of Respiratory Critical Care Medicine* 152: 977–83.

Tengs TO, Osgood ND (2001) The link between smoking and impotence: two decades of evidence. *Preventive Medicine* 32(6): 447–52.

Thyrian JR, Hannöver W, Grempler J *et al.* (2006) An intervention to support postpartum women to quit smoking or remain smoke-free. *Journal of Midwifery and Women's Health* 51: 45–50.

Tuthill DR, Stewart JH, Coles EC *et al.* (1999) Maternal cigarette smoking and pregnancy outcome. *Paediatric and Perinatal Epidemiology* 13(3): 245–53.

Twigg L, Moon G, Walker S (2004) The smoking epidemic in England. Health Development Agency. www.publichealth.nice.org.uk (Accessed: 4/12/2005).

US Public Health Service (1980) The health consequences of smoking for women: a report of the Surgeon General. Washington DC, Office of the Assistant Secretary for Health Office on Smoking and Health, US Public Health Service.

West R, McNeill A, Raw M (2000) Smoking cessation guidelines for health professionals: An update. *Thorax* 55: 987–99.

West R, Raw M (2002) *Meeting Department of Health smoking cessation targets: recommendations for primary care trusts and practitioners.* Health Development Agency.

White P, Watt J (2002) *Tobacco in London: Facts and Issues.* London, SmokeFree London. www.smokefreelondon.org/ (accessed 4/12/06).

Wiemann CM, Berenson AB, San-Miguel VV (1994) Tobacco, alcohol and illicit drug use among pregnant women. Age and racial/ethnic differences. *Journal of Reproductive Medicine* 39(10): 769–76.

Wilkinson D, Abraham C (2004) Constructing an integrated model of the antecedents of adolescent smoking. *British Journal of Health Psychology* 9(3): 315–33.

Chapter 4
Teenage Pregnancy: Everyone's Business

Vanessa Hollings, Claire Jackson and Clare McCann

> In the world's richest nations, more than three-quarters of a
> million teenagers will become mothers in the next twelve months
> (UNICEF 2001)

Introduction

Teenage pregnancy rates in the UK are amongst the highest in
Western Europe, and are considered to be of such concern that in
1999 the Government established a dedicated Teenage Pregnancy
Unit with the aim of reducing the under-18 conception rate and
supporting teenage parents. The Department for Education and
Skills recognises the social impact of teenage pregnancy and parenthood, and in their guidance to local authorities they highlight
the evidence that suggests that having children at a young age
can damage young women's health and well-being (DfES 2006).
Young parents possess the ability to become competent parents,
however, the evidence is clear that children born to teenage parents are at increased risk of experiencing adverse health and social
outcomes in later life (Swann *et al.* 2003). A debate exists as to
whether or not teenage pregnancy is a public health issue (Bailey
2005), and whether the adverse outcomes experienced by some
teenage mothers and their babies are causally related to the age of
the mother or other factors.

The pregnant teenager faces three main choices:

- To continue with the pregnancy and keep the baby
- To continue with the pregnancy and elect to have the baby
  adopted
- To terminate the pregnancy

This chapter is dedicated to the mothers who wish to continue with their pregnancies. Midwives are in a prime position to work with young mothers, supported or not, to maximise health outcomes for both mother and baby. The chapter will examine the individual and population needs of young people who use maternity services, and make suggestions for the commissioning and delivery of appropriate and sensitive care.

Background

Teenage pregnancy is not a new phenomenon in the UK, although teenagers are far less likely to become pregnant now than they were in the early 1970s (Figures 4.1 and 4.2). The 1967 Abortion

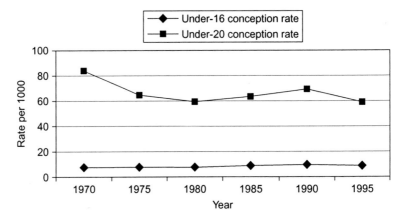

Figure 4.1 England teenage conception rates 1970–1995.
Source: Brook (2002) Factsheet 2.

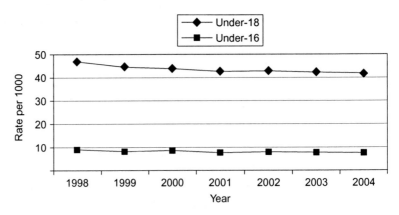

Figure 4.2 England teenage conception rates 1998–2004.
Source: Office for National Statistics/Teenage Pregnancy Unit (cited in DfES 2006).

Act led to a sharp decline in the proportion of young women choosing motherhood when the choice was offered to terminate unwanted pregnancies. The introduction of free contraception in 1974 resulted in a reduction in conceptions. However, fears in relation to confidentiality when accessing contraceptive services and cuts in those services, unemployment and lack of opportunities for young people have been identified as some of the reasons as to why teenage conception rates rose during the 1980s. In England and Wales, between 1990 and 1995, there was a 15% reduction in conceptions in young people aged 20 and under, which coincided with the increased provision of specialist young people's sexual health services by 33% during this time. The 1995 alert over the increased risk of deep vein thrombosis to those using third-generation contraceptive pills caused a significant increase in teenage conception rates (Brook 2002).

During the late 1990s, teenage conception rates continued on their downward trend, linked to strategies developed to reduce teenage pregnancies and improve sexual health (Brook 2002). Since the 1970s the conception rates for young women aged 16 and under have mirrored the rates of those aged 20 and under, although since 1998 the conception rate for those 16 and under has fallen more significantly than in older age groups of teenagers.

The Social Exclusion Unit (SEU) report on Teenage Pregnancy (1999) identified the UK teenage conception rates as being twice that of Germany and three times that of France. Although the rates vary widely across England (see Table 4.1) and Wales, teenage conception rates are higher in the North of England than the south (with the exception of London).

Table 4.1 Regional distribution of teenage pregnancies in the UK, 2001.

Region	Number of under-18 conceptions	Number of under-18 births
London	6201	2540
North East	2389	1502
Yorkshire and Humberside	4434	2723
West Midlands	4749	2641
North West	6020	3434
East Midlands	3076	1826
South West	3230	1743
South East	5022	2559
East of England	3308	1741
Total	**38 439**	**20 710**

Source: Teenage Pregnancy Unit (2003).

Who becomes a pregnant teenager?

Ambition, aspiration, educational attainment and school enjoyment are contributing factors to early sexual activity and parenthood, whether planned or otherwise. In the UK, girls and young women from social class V are at approximately 10 times the risk of becoming teenage mothers as girls from social class I (Swann *et al.* 2003). In this report the authors describe the lack of clarity as to what extent the effects of teenage pregnancy are determined or mediated by poverty. Gold *et al.* (2002) examined the relationship between teen birth, income inequality and social capital in the United States. The findings provide evidence of adverse effects of poverty and income inequality in this client group, which manifested itself through social mistrust and lack of community participation. Furthermore, the exclusion of community 'norms' and activities may be a prediction for young parenthood, in addition to increasing exclusion from social and financial community level resources (Swann *et al.* 2003).

Studies have identified social deprivation as the key factor in the variation of abortion rates in the UK; young people from more affluent areas access termination of pregnancy more readily than teenagers from poorer backgrounds (SEU 1999). In their systematic review of the evidence, Swann *et al.* (2003) found that some young people were more at risk than others of becoming teenage parents if they were:

- Below average educational achievement at ages 7 and 16 years of age
- Socially and economically deprived
- Looked-after children or care leavers (2.5 times more at risk of becoming a teenage mother 18–24 months after leaving care)
- Homeless young people
- Excluded, underperforming or truanting from school
- Children of teenage mothers
- From some ethnic minority groups, particularly Bangladeshi, African Caribbean and Pakistani
- Involved in crime
- Misusing alcohol or drugs

Conception rates are slightly higher in the North of England than the South, although there is some regional variation. Where young women experience multiple risk factors, their likelihood of teenage parenthood increases exponentially.

Being a mother in teenage years

Teenage parenthood is perceived to be both a cause and consequence of social exclusion. Teenage parents are more likely to be unemployed, live in poverty, and to give birth to low birth-weight babies, who as toddlers are likely to be at increased risk of childhood accidents (SEU 1999). This link with social exclusion means that teenage parents are themselves likely to be in poorer health, have poorer access to health and social support and experience poorer health outcomes for themselves and their babies. While some teenagers view their pregnancy as positive and fulfilling, others reveal negative consequences (SEU 1999). Research reveals (Swann *et al.* 2003) that young parents experience poorer health and social outcomes, which is linked to inadequate access to appropriate care and support. These factors include:

Health	Negative short-, medium- and long-term health and mental health outcomes for young mothers.
Education	As well as being more likely to have problems at school before they become pregnant, young mothers are less likely to complete their education, have no qualifications and have lower income than their peers.
Housing	80% of under-18 mothers live in someone else's household and are more likely to have to move house during pregnancy.
Birthweight	Babies born to teenage mothers have lower birthweight, but this is likely to be linked to smoking, nutritional status and deprivation rather than age (DfES 2006).
Infant mortality	60% higher than for babies of older women (DfES 2006).
Mental health	Teenage mothers have three times higher the rate of postnatal depression of older mothers and a higher risk of poor mental health for three years after the birth (DfES 2006).
Feeding	Teenage mothers are less likely to breastfeed their babies (Botting *et al.* 1998).
Accidents	Children of teenage mothers are more likely to suffer accidents, especially poisoning or burns, and twice as likely to be admitted to

	hospital as a result of an accident or gastroenteritis (Peckham 1993).
Single parenthood	Children of teenage mothers are more likely to have the experience of being a lone-parent family and are generally at increased risk of poverty, poor housing, poor health and have lower rates of economic activity as adults (DfES 2006).
Family history	Daughters of teenage mothers may be more likely to become teenage mothers themselves (Berrington *et al.* 2005).

While there is little information on the outcomes for teenage fathers they seem to be similar to young mothers.

What about teenage fathers?

The Home Office Family Policy Unit (1998) promoted the strengthening of relationships between parents and sons, in particular the bond between fathers and sons. More recently, the National Service Framework (DoH 2004b) supports a cultural shift in all service provision, to include fathers in all aspects of a child's well-being. As with young mothers, young fathers are also at increased risk of emotional and relationship problems, particularly amongst those separated from their children (Department of Health, Social Services and Public Safety 2002). Young men may be reluctant to attend traditional parentcraft sessions due to fear of being judged; lack of support to attend from family and peers; reaction against authority and feeling out of place amongst a group of older parents. In one recent study healthcare professionals were found to know little about teenage fathers, did not see them as central to their task and felt they lacked the skills to engage with young men (Quinton, Pollock and Golding 2002). The Teenage Pregnancy Strategy (SEU 1999) identified specific actions to support the needs of boys and young men. This included targeted campaign materials and sexual health messages which meet their particular needs. The *Sexual Health and HIV Strategy* (DoH 2001) identifies that the particular needs of boys and young men should be taken into account in service development and sexual health education. Some would argue that there is an absence of gender-related targets in terms of health, which does not encourage health providers to focus specifically on men's health (Working with Young Men 2003).

Teen pregnancy good or bad? Midwives and the media

Teenage mothers see pregnancy as a 'career move'
(The Independent 2006)

The media have become increasingly interested in – and an influence on – teenage pregnancy. The above newspaper headline was reporting on a study of 41 mothers and 10 fathers, where participants revealed they often chose pregnancy as a positive move to enhance their future. They felt that becoming a parent was a way out of hardship and unhappiness, and offered them an opportunity for independence: an alternative to poorly paid employment with limited education and training options (Cater and Coleman 2006). This positive focus for young parents was reported negatively in the article headline, which increases potential for further prejudices in society.

Shakespeare (2004) explored the attitudes of midwives in relation to teenage pregnancy, and describes how participants in her study believed teenage mothers became pregnant intentionally. The underlying reasons for the pregnancy, midwives believed, included benefits, housing, and the provision of 'something to love'. The attitude of all healthcare workers who come into contact with young people is of vital importance, as young people often perceive health staff as unsympathetic and dismissive – clearly not an acceptable approach and one that is linked to a possible increase in non-attendance for maternity care.

Government strategies linked to teenage pregnancy

There is a plethora of policy drivers and key performance targets for both NHS organisations and local authority children's services that relate indirectly and directly to delivery of accessible and appropriate midwifery services for young people. These include:

The Health of the Nation: a Strategy for Health (DoH 1992) was the first national strategy to identify teenage pregnancy as an issue, and highlighted the importance of effective provision of contraceptive services for those people who wanted them. The document set a target to reduce the number of unwanted pregnancies in all age groups (DoH 1992).

The Teenage Pregnancy Strategy (SEU 1999) was introduced nationally in 1999 following a report from the Social Exclusion Unit, bringing teenage pregnancy into a higher political arena. The report identified the key risk factors associated with teenage pregnancy and teenage parenthood, and established two clear targets:

- To reduce the rate of under-18 conceptions by 50% by 2010 and set a firmly established downward trend in conception rates for under-16s by 2010
- To achieve a reduction in the risk of long-term social exclusion faced by teenage parents and their children

A later target was introduced increasing the numbers of teenage mothers engaged in employment, education and training to 60% by 2010.

The Teenage Pregnancy Strategy emphasised the importance of partnership working and provided funding to local areas through the introduction of local implementation grants, with the aim to develop local action plans and employ specific teenage pregnancy co-ordinators. Local action plans were developed to reflect the national plan and focused on four key evidence-based areas:

- Media and communication
- Better prevention: sex and relationship education
- Better prevention: services
- Better support for teenage parents

The Teenage Pregnancy Unit was established as a cross-government initiative to support the strategy, through regional and local teenage pregnancy co-ordinators. It also produced a range of guidance, research and statistical briefings, including a guide to commissioning and delivering maternity services for young parents.

Tackling Health Inequalities (DoH 2003) highlighted the importance of engagement of communities and individuals to reduce health inequalities and promote health and well-being, in recognition that individuals or populations have a greater idea of what can work best for them in their particular circumstances. This philosophy can be used when working with young people, and is described later in this chapter. Peer support has been highlighted as an effective way of engaging and supporting teenage parents (Shakespeare 2004).

Choosing Health: Making Healthy Choices Easier (DoH 2004c) This government White Paper broadened the teenage conception target to include the improvement of sexual health and made further links to the health of teenage parents and their children. They included:

- To reduce the under-18 conception rate by 50% by 2010 (from the 1998 baseline) as part of the broader strategy to improve sexual health
- Reduce health inequalities by 10% by 2010 as measured by infant mortality and life expectancy at birth.

This strategy proposes the introduction of screening for *Chlamydia*, a common sexually transmitted infection, to 15–24 year olds from 2006, and enhanced access to community-based sexual health services.

Sure Start and Sure Start Plus The introduction of Sure Start local programmes targeted the 20% most deprived neighbourhoods throughout England to combine nursery education, family support, employment advice, childcare and health services on one site. The Sure Start approach is now being extended and mainstreamed through a national network of children's centres. Around the country many maternity services and primary care trusts have worked with their local Sure Start programmes to raise the quality of maternity services for vulnerable women, including teenagers, by helping services develop in disadvantaged areas, while providing financial help to enable parents to afford quality childcare.

The Sure Start Plus teenage pregnancy pilot programme offered personal advisor support to pregnant young women and teenage mothers and fathers in 20 pilot areas, covering 35 local authorities. The advisor's role was to help young people make decisions about their pregnancy and future contraception and provide a co-ordinated package of support for teenage parents to help improve their health outcomes and enable them to continue their education and training.

A number of Sure Start Plus programmes also funded specialist midwifery and health visitor posts to deliver young-people-friendly antenatal group work and individual support to young parents. Recommendations from the evaluation of these pilots has been integrated into National Children's Centre guidance.

Every Child Matters: Change for Children (DfES 2004) set out five key outcomes to improve the life chances of children and young people. They are:

- Being healthy, including sexually healthy
- Staying safe including safe from sexual exploitation

- Enjoying and achieving
- Making a positive contribution
- Achieving economic well-being.

Children, Young People and Maternity National Service Framework (DoH 2004b) set out a 10-year strategy to improve health services and make them more tailored and inclusive for children, young people and pregnant women.

Module 11 sets standards for maternity services to be supportive and of high quality, designed around the individual needs of those using them, especially women who are vulnerable such as teenage parents. This standard includes reference to *Teenage Parents: Who Cares?* A guide to commissioning and delivering maternity services for young parents (DoH 2004a), which directs primary care trusts, maternity services, local authorities and other agencies to work together to deliver appropriate care for teenage parents.

Reduction of teenage conceptions is one of the key health targets for which local strategic partnerships (LSPs) are held responsible in their community plans or local area agreements (LAA). These are subject to formal performance management by regional government offices as part of the accreditation procedure for LSPs.

Teenage Pregnancy Next Steps: Guidance for Local Authorities and Primary Care Trusts on Effective Delivery of Local Strategies (DfES 2006) provided an update on progress of the initial Teenage Pregnancy Strategy. The document set out the findings of 'deep dive' reviews, which identified the key features of effective teenage pregnancy strategies. In areas where rates had reduced significantly their experience was compared and contrasted with what was happening in statistically similar areas, where rates were static or increasing. The successful local areas were characterised by the following factors, which confirm the evidence base of the strategy:

- Active engagement of all the key agencies who have a role in reducing teenage pregnancies
- A strong senior champion who was accountable for and took the lead in driving forward the strategy
- The existence of a discrete, credible, highly visible, young-people-friendly sexual health/contraceptive advice service, with a focus on health promotion as well as reactive services
- Strong delivery of sex and relationship education/personal social and health education by schools

- Targeted work with at-risk groups of young people, in particular looked-after children
- The availability and consistent take-up of sex and relationship education (SRE) training for professionals in partner organisations working with the most vulnerable young people
- A well resourced youth service, with a clear remit to tackle big social issues, such as young people's sexual health

This document reiterated the links to teenage pregnancy and deprivation and highlighted the range of other factors, in particular poor educational attainment and low aspiration, as having an impact over and above deprivation levels. To make a lasting and positive impact on teenage pregnancy rates, the document calls for the 'deep dive' findings to be implemented and embedded in children and young people's plans.

Commissioning maternity services for pregnant teenagers and young parents

Midwives and other healthcare professionals in the UK have never been in a better position to influence how services are delivered. National strategy documents highlighted earlier can be used in conjunction with local needs assessments as levers when developing proposals to initiate and/or mainstream midwifery programmes of care for teenage parents.

Commissioning of services is a statutory function of the primary care trusts (PCTs) that serve each local population. They 'buy' health services such as maternity care, and expect high standards and efficiency in return. It is important that midwives are fully aware of the commissioning process, especially when they want to make changes based on expressed need and evidence.

Commissioners and providers of maternity services should work collaboratively to ensure services delivered for young people are accessible and appropriate to meet their needs (TPU 2004). *Teenage Parents: Who Cares?* (DoH 2004a) suggests this is done by asking several questions:

- What is the percentage of teenagers who book late for antenatal care?
- What is the vaginal delivery rate among teenagers compared to the rest of the childbearing population?
- What is the rate of caesarean section among teenagers compared to the rest of the childbearing population?

- What is the incidence of low birthweight among teenage mothers?
- Can you identify the rate of postnatal depression among teenage mothers?
- What is the percentage of teenagers who initiate breastfeeding and are still breastfeeding at six weeks?
- What is the incidence of babies of teenagers admitted to hospital during their first year?
- What is the likelihood of pregnant teenagers returning to education, training or work?

Commissioning exists at various levels – as well as dealing with the short- and long-term needs of individuals and whole populations. The Audit Commission has argued that commissioning is a strategic activity, which should shape the market of care to meet future needs. Therefore commissioning, by its very nature, is concerned with change in the provision of care services. Commissioning must result in changes in the way frontline services are delivered. The commissioning process can most conveniently be thought of as a cycle (Figure 4.3).

Stage 1 of the commissioning process must be to identify the level of need in the locality, and this will be assisted by involving the community as described in Chapter 1 and below.

As already demonstrated, the health and social outcomes for young parents are significantly worse than for the rest of the population. However, there is no biological reason associated with age to indicate that outcomes for young people should not be good, and it appears to be linked to three other main factors:

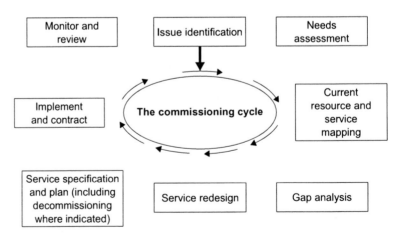

Figure 4.3 The commissioning cycle.

- Socioeconomic factors
- Educational attainment
- Access to appropriate care and support.

It is important to emphasise that young people are individuals, and not a homogenous group. They come from a wide variety of backgrounds; cultural, economic and religious. It is not possible or practical to place teenagers together with a 'label'; they are a group of individuals who will have their own unique set of circumstances and associated needs. Some may be pregnant in the context of a planned decision within a stable relationship with supportive family and friends, while others may find themselves very much alone with an unplanned and unwanted pregnancy. Services must be designed and delivered to meet this diversity of need.

Needs assessment

The needs assessment is the largest and most important element of the commissioning cycle as it is against these identified needs that services will be designed and ultimately delivered. A whole systems approach to needs assessment is essential; young people will not only have needs relating directly to their pregnancy or impending parenthood, but will often have needs across a wide spectrum. It is important that all aspects of young people's lives are considered, if organisations are to achieve objectives set out in *Every Child Matters: Change for Children* outcome framework (DfES 2004).

Service design

Once the level of need has been established the next crucial issue to consider is the service design and how it can take precedence alongside other service priorities to achieve sustained funding. How can maternity services for young people compare with cancer targets and the achievement of the 18-week waiting target? Knowing the level of need will help direct the service required.

- Do the numbers and level of need justify a dedicated team delivering services for young people?
- How can the services be integrated with mainstream services across agencies?

- Where will the service be delivered from to ensure it is accessible and appropriate to meet the needs of young people?

The funding attached to the Teenage Pregnancy Strategy (TPU 1999) has facilitated the development of innovative services to support teenage parents. The funding has enabled commissioners and providers to adopt a flexible approach to service development and take some calculated risks using a 'sounds good – let's do it' approach. However, the time comes with all short-term funding when it is necessary to evaluate initiatives objectively and establish which have been most effective in meeting the needs of the target population.

When considering development of maternity service models, providers must ensure their proposal is realistic and incorporates a system that guarantees resources are being targeted at those young people who are in greatest need. For example, a one-to-one caseload midwifery model may be suggested for all pregnant teenagers with the evidence that this will best meet their needs, build confidence, rapport and communication and ultimately deliver improved outcomes for parent(s) and child. But when this is related back to the identified needs, can such a model be truly justified? Those more mature resourceful young people in a stable relationship with supportive family and friends may not require such intense support; a well-informed mainstream midwifery team may meet their needs.

Good practice tip: developing new services

- What are the needs of young people locally?
- What do you currently do?
- How much of it do you do?
- Why are you doing it?
- How are you doing it?
- Where is it currently done?
- Who does it?
- Is the new service value for money? Is it efficient?
- Will the service be of a high quality?

This commissioning approach fits well with the overall children's services agenda of developing staged services, universal, targeted and specialist support to meet individual need. Services need to work in partnership with other agencies e.g. social services, Connexions, youth offending teams, to help identify those young people who require specialist support and/or to develop criteria locally for levels of service available.

```
Good practice tip

All Tier 1 local authorities are required to have a Single Children's Plan
in place by March 2006. Make sure you are aware of the targets in your
local plan and, if possible, influence the content to include teenage
pregnancy and meeting the needs of teenage parents.
```

Involving young people

As outlined in Chapter 1, the importance of working in partnership with those who use health and social care services is paramount to maximising opportunities for health gain. The government report *Saving Lives: Our Healthier Nation* (DoH 1999:8) proposed a 'new three-way partnership comprising of individuals, communities, government', encouraging all three parties to work in unison to improve public health across all sections of society. Since then, most government health policy has encouraged service user involvement in health service planning and delivery. In particular, there is a drive for children and young people to have more opportunities to get involved in the design, provision and evaluation of policies and services that affect them or which they use (Children and Young People's Unit (CYPU) 2001).

Children and young people have a right to participate fully (Save the Children Fund (SCF) 1996; Sex Education Forum (SEF) 2003) and professionals have a responsibility to facilitate this participation. The benefits of this rights-based approach are that children and young people can become active in the participation process rather than merely consumers of a service (Baker 1996, Connexions Service National Unit (CSNU) 2002). For a convincing argument for involving young people, much can be learnt from the private sector that has engaged with young people to promote their goods for many years (Cutler 2002). Global corporations like Nike and McDonalds have long since learned that they can most effectively ascertain the needs, wants and desires of young people by involving them fully at the start and then engaging with them throughout the product development process.

An example of involvement/participation for young people is peer support or peer education.

Examples of good practice: peer education

Young people were recruited from a local area and undertook a comprehensive training and accreditation programme. Peer educators and volunteers were then attached to youth and community centres across the borough to undertake project work focusing on young people and sexual health.

The benefits for peer educators when participating in peer education programmes have been highlighted and include increased knowledge and ability, increased confidence, maturity, development of communication and inter personal skills (SEF 1999; DoH 2002; Peer Support Forum (PSF) 2001).

There are other ways of involving teenagers. For example, if services want to relocate into children's centres, midwives should consult with young people on their views of existing provision and any barriers to access. This can be supported by visiting a range of venues to identify which are the most acceptable. This consultation process must be cyclical, with midwives feeding information to colleagues, other service providers and ensuring feedback to young people.

Examples of good practice: involving teenagers

A booklet for teenage parents was designed by a teenage mother in conjunction with maternity services and funded through external partners. The booklet was piloted in one borough, and then rolled out across East Lancashire. The resource was targeted at young women who had a positive pregnancy test and aims to outline young people's choices and signpost them to appropriate support services. The booklet has been very successful and is now in its third edition. It was cited as 'gold standard' by the Teenage Pregnancy Unit.

Think about:

- How can midwives effectively involve young mothers and fathers in the development of maternity service provision?
- How can the views of young mothers and fathers be effectively represented to Commissioners?

Midwifery support: specialist or mainstream?

As previously detailed, UK national directives are clear that additional input into the care of teenagers is essential, when aiming to maximise health and social gain for the young mother and her child. Since the publication of the Teenage Pregnancy report (SEU 1999), many specialist midwifery roles have been developed (Byrom 2001; Perrow 2004; Mead *et al.* 2005, Wiggins *et al.* 2005), and are providing additional support and leadership in this area. Additionally, two specialist teenage pregnancy midwives established a national midwifery support network (TPU 2006), providing online support for midwives who work with teenage parents or have an interest in teenage pregnancy. Many providers and commissioners of maternity services are currently striving to mainstream support for teenagers, as it is recognised that specialist support, while essential, can not always address all the needs of young parents all of the time. In addition to this, teenage mothers and fathers come into contact with many other health professionals, who may need mentorship and training to assist with understanding the needs of this client group.

It would seem most appropriate to provide a combination of targeted and mainstream support, dependent on need, and midwives should think about the vulnerability of young people, and focus care accordingly. However, midwives cannot expect to provide all the support for teenage parents. As described in Chapter 1, working with a public health philosophy does not imply expansion of the midwife's role overall, but involves thinking laterally and linking effectively with relevant stakeholders in health and social care. Midwives should be aware of a full range of services in their local area so they can signpost young people to them for further information, support and advice, e.g. Connexions, benefits advice, sexual health services, housing, domestic abuse helplines, colleges and other training providers.

The poor outcomes of teenage birth may be the result of substandard care in pregnancy (SEU 1999). Raatikainen *et al.* (2005) undertook a study in Finland to examine the effect of self-defined 'high quality' maternity care on the outcomes for teen mothers and their babies. The study concluded that increased risks may be overcome with good care that is free and accessible. Antenatal care schemes that include social and behavioural services in addition to medical care have been shown to improve outcomes for teen mothers and their babies (Scholl *et al.* 1994).

Midwives have a prominent role to play in children's services and as such need also to consider where their services are being delivered. Clinical settings or GP surgeries may not be the most appropriate venue to see young people. There is a clear message across children's services that maternity care should be integrated and delivered from venues specifically developed for children and young people e.g. integrated children's centres, extended schools, youth centres etc. The provision of care in this way is part of the key delivery mechanisms to achieve the *Every Child Matters* (DfES 2004) outcomes, and to maximise opportunities for joint delivery of services, health promotion work and the promotion of other services available at the centre.

The midwife and the teenage parent

Global and national evidence suggests that pregnant teenagers, teenage parents and their children are at increased risk of poorer health and social outcomes. Significant challenges remain to achieve national targets and further reduce the risk of social exclusion for pregnant teenagers and young parents. It has been highlighted previously that not all teenage parents are vulnerable and in need of extra support. It may not be the age of the teenager that places them in a vulnerable position, but the fact that they could already be living in social isolation or in poverty.

In her study on the effects of poverty and motherhood, Hunt (2001) describes the negative attitudes of midwives, and how it was this fact alone that marginalised women who were disadvantaged. Individual attitudes of healthcare workers is the most important factor to consider when connecting with or caring for all mothers and fathers, particularly teenagers. As detailed in Chapter 1, midwives need to try understand the causes and reasons for the life choices people make, and that includes teenagers choosing to become parents. They need to feel safe, respected and valued so they can have confidence in health professionals (Wray 2005). Young people also need to be sure that services will be confidential, as sharing information about them to parents and other professionals is often their biggest fear. A negative experience with a midwife or other healthcare worker has the potential to destroy trust during the childbirth continuum, which could lead to a lack of desire to access care. A positive, nurturing relationship between the young parents and their midwife holds the potential to make a difference to two lives.

Midwives throughout the UK appear to be making a difference to the lives of young mothers and fathers, and in some instances the midwife is viewed as a role model for the teenage mother.

Their influence is such that in an evaluation of Sure Start Plus programmes in the UK, many young mothers expressed a wish to become midwives themselves (Wiggins *et al.* 2005). Above all, midwives need to understand the often complex and challenging lives of some teenagers and other vulnerable women if they are to make a significant difference in influencing the future.

> ...midwives should try to remember that women from disadvantaged groups are human beings first, disadvantaged second
>
> (Hunt 2001:76)

Key implications for midwifery practice

- Develop and deliver specific training and awareness raising for midwives and student midwives.
- Develop youth-centred groups offering support on health, benefits, social care, housing and employment, education and training opportunities.
- Devise a 'making decisions' contact sheet for all midwifery staff using the *Every Child Matters* outcomes headings and detailing support services in your area.
- Involve young people by asking their views, and then making recommendations.
- Recognise the importance of peer support.
- Make midwifery services accessible to young people through the use of community venues (e.g. children's centres).
- Acknowledge the need to support young parents to make choices about future contraception.
- Offer information on accessible, youth-friendly services following birth.
- Acknowledge the need to work with partner agencies to identify the needs of young fathers to encourage them to engage and form positive relationships with their babies.

References

Bailey P (2005) Teenage pregnancies: is the high rate of teenage pregnancy and parenthood in the UK a public health problem? *Journal of Family Planning and Reproductive Health Care* 31(4): 315–19.

Baker J (1996) *The Fourth Partner: Participant or Consumer*. Leicester, Youth Work Press.

Berrington A, Diamond I, Ingham R *et al.* (2005) *Consequences of Teenage Motherhood: pathways which minimise the long-term negative impacts of teenage childbearing.* University of Southampton.

Botting B, Rosato M, Wood R (1998) Teenage mothers and the health of their children. *Population Trends* 93: 19–28.

Brook (2002) *Factsheet 2: Teenage Conceptions: Statistics and Trends, April 2002.* Brook, London.

Byrom S (2001) Supporting teenage parents. In English National Board (2001) *Midwives in Action: a resource.* London, ENB.

Cater S, Coleman L (2006) 'Planned' Teenage Pregnancy. *Perspectives of Young Parents from Disadvantaged Backgrounds.* Joseph Rowntree Foundation. Bristol, Policy Press.

Children and Young People's Unit (2001) *Building A Strategy For Children and Young People.* London, Children and Young People's Unit.

Connexions Service National Unit (2002) *Putting Young People First.* Nottingham, Department for Education and Skills.

Cutler D (2002) *Taking The Initiative.* London, Children and Young People's Unit.

Department for Education and Skills (2004) *Every Child Matters: Change for Children.* London, The Stationery Office. www.dfes.gov.uk/everychildmatters/ (accessed 4/12/06).

Department for Education and Skills (2006) *Teenage Pregnancy Next Steps: Guidance for Local Authorities and Primary Care Trusts on Effective Delivery of Local Strategies.* London, DfES Publications.

Department of Health (1992) *The Health of the Nation.* London, The Stationery Office.

Department of Health (1999) *Saving Lives: Our Healthier Nation.* London, The Stationery Office.

Department of Health (2001) *The National Strategy for Sexual Health and HIV.* London, The Stationery Office.

Department of Health (2002) *Listening, Hearing and Responding.* London, Department of Health Publications.

Department of Health (2003) *Tackling Health Inequalities: a Programme for Action.* London, The Stationery Office.

Department of Health (2004a) *Teenage Parents: Who Cares?: a guide to commissioning and delivering maternity services for young parents.* London, the Stationery Office.

Department of Health (2004b) *National Service Framework for Children, Young People and Maternity Services.* London, The Stationery Office.

Department of Health (2004c) *Choosing Health: Making Healthy Choices Easier.* London, The Stationery Office.

Department of Health, Social Services and Public Safety (2002) *Teenage Pregnancy and Parenthood: strategy and action plan 2002–2007.* Belfast. www.dhsspsni.gov.uk/teenagepregnancy-action0207.pdf#search=%22 (Working%20Group%20on%20Teenage%20Pregnancy%20%26%20 Parenthood%202000).%22 (accessed 5/12/06).

Gold R, Kennedy B, Connell F, Kawachi I (2002) Teen births, income inequality and social capital: developing an understanding of the causal pathway. *Health and Place* 8(2): 77–83.

Goodchild S, Owen J (2006) *Teenage mothers see pregnancy as a 'career move'. The Independent* 16 July 2006. http://news.independent.co.uk/uk/this_britain/article1180248.ece accessed 5/12/06.

Home Office Policy Unit (1998) *Boys, Young Men and Fathers: a ministerial seminar.* 16th November 1998. www.nationalarchives.gov.uk/ERO/records/ho415/1/cpd/fmpu/boys.htm (accessed 5/12/06).

Hunt S (2001) Tackling disadvantage in maternity care. In English National Board (2001) *Midwives in Action.* London, ENB.

Mead M, Brooks F, Windle K *et al.* (2005) Evaluation of a midwifery support service for pregnant teenagers *British Journal of Midwifery* 13(12): 762–66.

Peckham S (1993) Preventing unplanned teenage pregnancies. *Public Health* 107: 125–33.

Peer Support Forum (2001) *Different Models of Peer Support.* www.mentalhealth.org.uk/welcome/ (accessed 13/12/05).

Perrow F (2004) Investing in teenage parents: what maternity services can do. *RCM Journal* 7(6): 250–51.

Quinton D, Pollock S, Golding J (2002) *The Transition to Fatherhood in Young Men: Influences on Commitment Youth.* Citizenship and Social Change Programme, Sheffield.

Raatikainen K, Heiskanen N, Verkasalo PK, Seppo H (2005) Good outcome of teenage pregnancies in high-quality care. *European Journal of Public Health* 16(2) 157–61.

Save The Children Fund (1996) *Children's Participation Pack.* London, SCF.

Scholl TO, Hediger ML, Belsky DH (1994) Prenatal care and maternal health during adolescent pregnancy: a review and meta-analysis. *Journal of Adolescent Health* 15: 444–56.

Sex Education Forum (1999) Peer education approaches to sex and relationships education. *Forum Factsheet* 20. www.ncb.org.uk (accessed 13/12/06).

Sex Education Forum (2003) Sex and Relationships Education Framework. *Forum Factsheet 30.* www.ncb.org.uk (accessed 13/12/06).

Shakespeare D (2004) Exploring midwives' attitudes to teenage pregnancy. *British Journal of Midwifery* 12(5): 320–27.

Social Exclusion Unit (1999) *Teenage Pregnancy: Report by the Social Exclusion Unit.* London, The Stationery Office.

Swann C, Bowe K, McCormick G, Kosmin M (2003) *Teenage Pregnancy and Parenthood: A review of reviews.* Evidence Briefing, Health Development Agency. London, Sure Start. www.nice.org.uk/page.aspx?o=502529 (accessed 11/12/06).

Teenage Pregnancy Unit (2001) *A Guide to Involving Young People in Teenage Pregnancy Work.* London, TPU. www.dfes.gov.uk/teenagepregnancy/dsp_content.cfm?pageid=112 (accessed 13/12/06).

Teenage Pregnancy Unit (2004) *Teenage Parents: Who Cares? A guide to commissioning and delivering maternity services for young parents.* London, TPU.

Teenage Pregnancy Unit (2006) Midwifery Network www.rcm.org.uk/professional/pages/practice.php?id=6 (accessed 13/12/06).

UNICEF (2001) A league table of teenage births in rich nations. *Innocenti Report Card* No.3, Florence, Innocenti Research Centre.

Wiggins M, Rosat M, Austerberry H *et al.* (2005) *Sure Start Plus National Evaluation: final report.* Social Science Research Unit, Institute of Education, University of London.

Working with Young Men (January 2003) *Young Men on the Margins: Strategies for Engagement.* WWYM Publications. www.workingwithmen/org/ (accessed 13/12/06).

Wray J (2005) Confidentiality and teenage pregnancy: the affinity gap *Midwives* 8(12): 493.

Chapter 5
Sexual Health: A Potential Time Bomb

Julie Kelly and Grace Edwards

> There is no part of the UK that is unaffected by HIV and other
> sexually transmitted infections
> > (Pat Troop, Chief Executive, Health Protection Agency, 2005)

Introduction

Sexual health is not just about infections. Sexual and reproductive
health has a profound effect on individuals, communities and
society. It is about unplanned pregnancies, the timing of which
may in turn affect social outcomes, financial potential and future
prospects. But there are also wider public health implications for
poor sexual health. The government's Public Health White Paper,
Choosing Health: Making Healthier Choices Easier (DoH 2004a) highlighted for the first time key priorities for action. These are:

- Reducing the numbers of people who smoke
- Reducing obesity and improving diet and nutrition
- Increasing exercise
- Encouraging and supporting sensible drinking
- Improving sexual health
- Improving mental health

Many of these issues have been addressed in previous chapters
and some aspects of sexual health have been explored in Chapter 4
in connection with teenage pregnancy. This chapter will concentrate on the wider implications of poor sexual health and discuss
some ways of addressing these issues.

What do we mean by sexual health and why is it so important?

The World Health Organization (WHO) working definition of sexual health is:

> A state of physical, emotional, mental and social wellbeing related to sexuality; not merely the absence of disease, dysfunction or infirmity. Sexual health requires a positive and respectful approach to sexuality and sexual relationships, as well as the possibility of having pleasurable and safe sexual experiences, free of coercion, discrimination and violence. For sexual health to be attained and maintained, the sexual rights of all persons must be protected, respected and fulfilled
>
> (WHO website)

There is a clear relationship between sexual ill health, poverty and social exclusion. Poor sexual health can be severely debilitating and some sexually transmitted infections, if left untreated, can have extremely serious consequences, e.g. the development of pelvic inflammatory disease, chronic abdominal pain, infertility and ectopic pregnancy.

Some groups in the UK are disproportionately affected by poor sexual health. They include women, young people, gay men and some black and minority ethnic communities. Sexual risk-taking is also increasing across the population and yet sexual health remains a stigmatised issue and levels of public awareness of the risks are low.

Sexual health and the inequalities associated with it are clearly a cause for public health concern, in relation to both the cost to the NHS and other services and to the health of our population. While there is a fairly limited evidence base in relation to the economics of sexual health, some studies have attempted to demonstrate the financial burden of poor sexual health in addition to the burden to the individual.

The Public Health Laboratory Service, Communicable Disease Surveillance Centre (PHLS–CDSC) published research in 2001 which estimated that the average lifetime treatment and care cost for a HIV-positive infected adult was between £135 000 and £181 000. However, this research also concluded that for every HIV infection that is prevented, the saving could be between £500 000 and £1 million over a lifetime. This figure includes additional costs to the economy, for example, hours lost from work (Health Protection Agency 2001).

The Health Protection Agency estimates that the yearly costs of treating sexually transmitted infections in the UK is over £700 million and this figure does not take into account the amount of money invested in treating illness that is a consequence of an undiagnosed infection, e.g. ectopic pregnancy or infertility.

The message is clear – prevention is better than cure. Prevention not only reduces the burden of ill health to the community but also to the NHS and the system. From a common sense health protection perspective, the fewer infected people there are, the smaller the risk of onward transmission to others.

There are strong arguments for investment in the prevention of sexually transmitted infections, and the same can also be said for investment in contraceptive services and access to contraception. In 2004 the Family Planning Association (fpa) estimated that there are big savings to be made by investing in contraception and estimated the cost to be £2.5 billion per year. Research also suggested that this figure could be increased significantly even further by revising the current supply of NHS contraceptive methods to better reflect what women prefer, and thus potentially leading to a reduction in the number of unplanned pregnancies and abortions. This research estimated that this could bring about an additional cost saving of up to £1 billion over 15 years (Armstrong *et al.* 2005).

Historical trends in sexual health

Discussions around sexual health are not new. Sefton (2001) described how it is widely accepted by historians that Columbus and his men brought syphilis back from the New World on their return to Europe in 1493. Famous victims of syphilis are said to include Ivan the Terrible, Henry VIII, Toulouse Lautrec, Randolph Churchill and Al Capone.

However, before the sexual revolution in the 1960s and 1970s the public were more concerned with pregnancy than sexually transmitted diseases.

The use of condoms was common and these were made from sheepskin, snakeskin, other animal intestines and later linen. Sometimes lemon juice and vinegar were added, which acted as a spermicide. Before the 20th century there was no understanding about vaginal pH, but users knew that this would prevent pregnancy.

Blacksmith (2000) described the discovery of the Ebers Papyrus (1550BC) where women were advised to grind together dates, acacia and honey into a moist paste, soak wool in the mixture and place in the vagina. This was apparently a very effective way to prevent pregnancy. Aristotle suggested soaking cotton in a mix of lemon, dried fish mixed with lemon and olive oil for use as a barrier method of contraception.

Coitus interruptus, the act of interrupting intercourse before the man had ejaculated, was as common in the past ages as it is today.

The sexual revolution in the 1960s and 1970s marked a new openness around sex and heralded a dramatic change in sexual health and sexual independence. Feminism was becoming established as women began to address some of the societal gender inequalities. The introduction of the contraceptive pill in 1960 gave women access to easy and reliable contraception and control of their own fertility. In this period before the advent of HIV and AIDS there were few concerns about sexual liberation. It is interesting that by the early 1980s women had established sexual behaviours similar to those of men. They had more partners (two to three times), starting at an earlier age (by three to five years), than women a decade earlier (Ridgeway 1997).

Recent UK trends in sexually transmitted infections

The rate at which sexually transmitted infections are rising in the UK is worrying. Diagnoses of sexually transmitted infections in the UK had fallen significantly in the mid to late 1980s. This was during the period following the much-publicised onset of the HIV and AIDS epidemic. The levels of sexually transmitted infections remained low until just after the mid-1990s. However, data collected from genitourinary medicine (GUM) clinics from 1996–2001 showed substantial increases in new diagnoses of infections. Almost all sexually transmitted infections have shown dramatic increases with over one million people attending GUM clinics each year (DoH 2000). The commonest infections include chlamydia, non-specific urethritis and wart virus infections. The concern is for those people who do not seek treatment or are unaware that they are infected. While the increase in new diagnoses gives health professionals clear cause for concern, we should remember that this data only includes those who have accessed services. As many sexually transmitted infections have no symptoms, the extent of the problem is likely to be much greater.

Chlamydia

A common example of an infection where many people are unaware they are infected is chlamydia, where levels of infection in the UK have more than doubled over the past 10 years, particularly in teenagers. In 2004, genital chlamydial infection remained the most common sexually transmitted infection diagnosed in GUM clinics in the UK. Chlamydia is a bacterial infection that can be treated and cured orally with antibiotics; however, it has no symptoms in at least 70% of women and 50% of men (HPA 2005).

Three-quarters of chlamydia diagnoses in women were in young women, and 56% of diagnoses in men were in young men (HPA 2005). The infection rate has been estimated at around 11% in women but worryingly, this infection is often asymptomatic and may not be diagnosed until fertility problems are apparent. If chlamydia is untreated, the consequences may be serious and include pelvic inflammatory disease, which can progress to ectopic pregnancy and infertility. Complications among men with untreated infection include urethritis, epididymitis and Reiter's syndrome (chlamydia-associated arthritis) (National Chlamydia Screening Programme 2005). Simms and Stephenson found evidence of chlamydia in around 40% of women who underwent laparoscopy for pelvic inflammatory disease much of which had not previously been suspected (Simms and Stephenson 2000).

HIV and AIDS

The number of people with HIV is also worrying. In 2004 there were an estimated 58 300 people living with HIV in the UK, of which an estimated 34% were unaware they had become infected. Although most midwives are familiar with dealing with women with HIV, it is worth revisiting how the infection is transmitted.

The human immunodeficiency virus (HIV) which causes acquired immunodeficiency syndrome (AIDS) is transmitted through body fluids, in particular blood, semen, vaginal secretions and breast-milk. One can become infected with HIV through:

- Unprotected sexual intercourse with an infected partner
- Sharing needles when injecting or other use of contaminated injection or other skin piercing equipment
- Blood and blood products, for example, infected transfusions and organ tissue transplants
- Transmission from infected mother to child in the womb or at birth and breastfeeding.

HIV weakens the human body's immune system, making it difficult to fight infection. Treatments exist which can prevent the onset of AIDS and although there are side effects, a person can lead a healthy active life with a long life expectancy if they respond well to treatment. However, they can still transmit the infection to others. Treatments do exist which can prevent the onset of AIDS and allow periods of illness to be followed by periods of remission. However, there is still no cure for AIDS. Research is currently under way into vaccines, but none is yet available (National AIDS Trust 2006).

In the UK, there has also been a year on year increase in the number of people who have become infected through heterosexual partners, suggesting that messages on HIV and sexually transmitted infections are being ignored (HPA 2005). According to figures published by the Health Protection Agency (2005) in 2004 approximately one in every 548 pregnant women in the UK was HIV-infected. Most cases were identified in women who themselves were born in high prevalence regions, particularly sub-Saharan Africa and Central America and the Caribbean. However, the prevalence of HIV among women born in the UK continues to rise slowly. As the AIDS epidemic continues, the total global population living with HIV and AIDS has grown to a staggering 40 million and the number of people who have lost their lives to the disease totals an estimated 30 million (HPA 2005).

If a pregnant woman has HIV but either does not disclose this or is unaware of her infection status, the risk of mother-to-child transmission of HIV is around 25%. However, if the woman receives anti-retroviral therapy during pregnancy, has a caesarean section and does not breastfeed, the risk of transmission falls to around 1% (National Study of HIV in Pregnancy and Childhood 2005). The National Study of HIV in Pregnancy and Childhood is a survey run by the Royal College of Obstetricians and Gynaecologists (RCOG) and the Royal College of Paediatrics and Child Health (RCPCH) to give intelligence surveillance on the rates of HIV infections in pregnancy and children. This data helps to inform government policy and practice around supporting women and their families who are HIV-positive.

Other sexually transmitted infections

Although over the past five years there has been an 11% decrease in the number of new cases of gonorrhoea reported, 42% of the cases in women were under the age of 20 (HPA 2005). However, despite this downturn, young people in the UK are disproportionately affected by gonorrhoea and also chlamydia (as discussed earlier) and genital warts. Rates of diagnoses continued to increase among young people in 2004, with the highest rates of gonorrhoea diseases seen among young men aged 20–24 (HPA 2005).

The trend is remarkably different for syphilis, which rose by 37% between 2003 and 2004 in the UK. However, 88% of all diagnoses were in men, of which more than half were in homosexual men. The rates were also higher in slightly older men with the highest rates found among men aged 25–34 and 35–44 (HPA 2005).

The most commonly diagnosed viral sexually transmitted infection is that of genital warts. Over the last few years, new diagnoses of genital warts rose by 4.2% (HPA 2005). Again the highest rates were seen in younger age groups, men aged 20–24 and – worryingly – young women aged 16–19. The prevalence of genital warts is likely to be vastly underestimated, as figures are only available for people who attend for treatment. Similar trends are apparent for genital herpes.

Recent UK trends in sexual activity and behaviours

The recent and continued increase in the diagnoses of new episodes of sexually transmitted infections in the UK and the high rates of teenage conceptions are an indication of an increase in sexual risk-taking behaviour among many population groups (Fenton and Hughes 2003). While the introduction of the National Chlamydia Screening Programme and encouragement for people to access testing and treatment services for sexually transmitted infection may have contributed to this increase in diagnoses, studies have shown a change in patterns of sexual behaviour in the UK.

The second National Survey of Sexual Attitudes and Lifestyles (NATSAL) (Erens *et al.* 2003) provides the most recent data on attitudes towards sex and sexuality and on patterns of sexual behaviours in Britain. In both men and women, the number of lifetime heterosexual partners has increased significantly between 1990 and 2000 with the average number of partners increasing from 8.6 to 12.7 and 3.7 to 6.5 in men and women respectively. Since 1990, the age at which young people have first intercourse has fallen, a larger proportion of people are having sex with multiple partners and a greater proportion of men are reporting having had sex with another man (Johnson *et al.* 2001). The issue of 'concurrency,' i.e. multiple partners, is of particular interest. The number of people reporting having had more than one partner at the same time has increased since 1990, which has implications for the increased likelihood of onward transmission of sexually transmitted infections as more people are being exposed. Again, the rate was higher among young people with 20% of young men and 15% of young women aged between 15–24 years having more than one partner at the same time in the past year.

Ellis *et al.* (2003) found that sexual behaviour may be influenced by a number of factors, including the following:

- Low self-esteem
- Lack of skills, e.g. how to use a condom
- Lack of negotiation skills e.g. how to say no to sex without a condom
- Lack of knowledge about the risks of different sexual behaviours
- Availability of contraceptives and access to services
- Peer pressure
- Attitudes and the stigmatisation of sexual health in society, which may affect people's willingness to access services.

Levels of awareness about sexually transmitted infections are also poor in the UK. A recently commissioned survey, which sought views from over 2000 people over the age of 15 (National AIDS Trust 2006) found that many of those who participated were not aware that HIV could be transmitted from one person to another through unprotected sex. Even more alarmingly, 15% of those surveyed said that they would never or rarely use a condom the first time they had sex with a new partner, with only 10% prepared to undergo testing for HIV before they stopped using a condom in a new relationship.

Sexual health, social class and deprivation

Being poor affects health. This concept has been explored in Chapters 1 and 2 and runs through many of the chapters of this book. Being poor also affects sexual health. There are proven links between social deprivation and sexually transmitted infections (STIs), abortions and teenage conceptions, with girls from the poorest backgrounds being 10 times more likely to become teenage mothers than girls from wealthier backgrounds.

One of the ultimate outcomes of poor sexual health is unplanned pregnancy, and this is particularly problematic for teenagers. Throughout the developed world, teenage pregnancy occurs most frequently among those young people who have been disadvantaged in childhood themselves. For example, they have grown up in poverty and have poor expectations of education and low aspirations in relation to employment (Botting *et al.* 1998). Teenage parents are far less likely to continue with their education and often come from the most deprived parts of the country. If you are a socially excluded teenager you are more likely to become a teenage parent and if you become a parent while in your teens, you are more likely to become socially excluded. The issue is both a cause and a symptom of social exclusion. Children born to teenage mothers generally face greater disadvantage than those born to older parents and are more likely to become teenage parents themselves, thus perpetuating the cycle of early parenthood and social exclusion (Department for Education and Skills 2006).

Although there is a great deal of work being undertaken around prevention and support for teenagers who become pregnant (see page 77 for national policy), the UK still has the highest rate of teenage pregnancy in Europe, with rates that are twice as high as Germany, three times as high as France and six times as high as the Netherlands (DoH 1999). Unintended pregnancies increase the risk of poor social, economic and health prospects for both mother and child. In 2003, 42 173 under 18-year-olds in the UK conceived. This equates to a rate of 42.3 conceptions per 1000 young women aged 15–17 in 2003. Approximately two-fifths of these pregnancies resulted in an abortion (Office for National Statistics 2005). Analysis has also highlighted that the younger a woman is, the more likely she is to have a termination. In 2002, 61% of conceptions to 14-year-olds resulted in legal abortions with 55% of 15-year-old girls opting to terminate their pregnancy (ONS 2004). These figures would suggest that pregnancy was unplanned and therefore sexual health may have been compromised in many cases. This idea is supported by research undertaken by the Health Education Authority, which suggested that there has been an increase in risky sexual behaviour, and that there is still ignorance about the possible consequences.

There has also been a noticeable drop in the age at which young people start having sex. Forty years ago, the average age at which people started having sex was 21. Today it is 17. Worryingly, between a third and a half of teenagers do not use contraception at first intercourse. Research by Dawe and Meltzer found that over a quarter of 14–15 year olds thought that the contraceptive pill protects against infection and most people questioned did not know what chlamydia was (Dawe and Meltzer 1999).

People of all ages from more deprived backgrounds are more likely to experience poor sexual health. The highest rates of sexually transmitted infections are found in women, particularly young women, gay men, teenagers, young adults and black and minority ethnic groups (Hughes *et al.* 2000). A recent summary factsheet on sexual health from the Department of Health (DoH 2006a) stated that sexually transmitted infections disproportionately affect young people and are more prevalent in deprived areas with poor educational attainment and low aspiration. The sheet also stated that people living in London are disproportionately affected by poor sexual health. HIV disproportionately affects young gay men (under 40); those with lower educational attainment; and those from black African communities.

It is well documented that those living in deprivation are more likely to experience lower levels of education attainment. A recent study by Rutherford *et al.* (2006) examined whether or not there are links between low levels of literacy and sexual behaviour and knowledge. Their study concluded that there is a link and moreover that those in the lower literacy group were significantly more likely to:

- have been under 16 years of age the first time they had sex
- be significantly less likely to know when the most fertile time is during the menstrual cycle
- be significantly less likely to be able to identify sexually transmitted infections
- be significantly less likely to be aware that infections can be transmitted through both oral and anal sex
- be more likely to have difficulties understanding health literature distributed in clinics.

Example of good practice

As part of the original Sure Start Plus project, Liverpool Women's NHS Foundation Trust seconded a midwife to support young women who became pregnant, working closely with the Teenage Pregnancy Co-ordinator, Sure Start Plus and Connexions. When the Sure Start Plus ended this post was mainstreamed by the Trust with some financial support from the Teenage Pregnancy Co-ordinator.

This midwife provides outreach support for all young pregnant women and their partners and families and includes teenage friends. She undertook her Family Planning Certificate and now offers the full range of contraceptive advice to extended groups. Working alongside a supportive consultant obstetrician, she administers long-acting reversible contraception (LARC), condoms and offers some screening options to young women. She also uses the opportunity to advise non-pregnant friends about safe sex and refers them for appropriate screening and contraception.

What is being done in the UK to improve sexual health?

The National Strategy for Sexual Health and HIV (DoH 2001) is the government's 10-year plan to improve sexual health. The first national strategy in the UK of its kind, with an explicit aim to improve sexual health, it made clear the links between poor sexual health, social exclusion and poverty. The national strategy aims to:

- improve sexual health services – both prevention and treatment and care services
- improve access to – and the availability of – appropriate information and support
- reduce health inequalities
- improve sexual health outcomes for all.

In 2004, the Department of Health produced an accompanying implementation action plan detailing how the evidence-based interventions in the strategy will be delivered at the national, regional and local levels (DoH, 2004b).

Another key policy driver for improvements in the sexual health of young people was the report *Teenage Pregnancy* (1999) produced on behalf of the government by the Social Exclusion Unit. The Social Exclusion Unit identified three key factors that contribute to high teenage conceptions: low expectations; ignorance about contraception, relationships, and what it means to be a parent; and mixed messages about sex.

The Social Exclusion Unit report identified four key areas for action:

- A national media campaign
- Joined-up action between health and local authorities
- Better prevention in schools, non-school settings and contraceptive services
- Better support for pregnant teenagers and teenage parents.

It also set out two key objectives for the national teenage pregnancy strategy:

- To halve the under-18 conception rate in England by 2010
- The participation of 60% of teenage parents in education, training or employment, to reduce the risk of their long-term social exclusion.

Every local authority has developed its own teenage pregnancy strategy, setting out how it will address the key areas for action, and contribute to the targets set out by the government.

The most recent key policy driver for change in relation to sexual health can be found in the government public health White Paper, *Choosing Health: Making Healthy Choices Easier* (2004) where it is cited as one of the top six priority areas for action. The White Paper reinforces previous strategic messages about sexual health improvement and also provides a focus for improving sexual health treatment and care through modernising services and improving access to them.

Choosing Health also came with an accompanying delivery plan, *Delivering Choosing Health: Making Healthy Choices Easier* (DoH 2004a). This document identified performance monitoring lines that primary care trusts (PCTs) would be measured against in their local delivery plans, which set out how a PCT will deliver on improving health. The monitoring lines are as follows:

- A reduction in the under-18 conception rate by 50% by 2010 as part of a broader strategy to improve sexual health
- 100% of patients' contacts in GUM clinics to be offered an appointment within 48 hours by 2008
- A decrease in the rates of new diagnoses of gonorrhoea by 2008
- An increase in the percentage of people aged 15 to 24 accepting chlamydia screening.

All of the above specifically refer to improving sexual health. There are also broader policy documents that impact on attempts to improve sexual health. They include:

- *Every Child Matters: Change for Children* (DfES 2004) – the key policy document for improving outcomes for children and young people which focuses on being healthy, staying safe, enjoying and achieving, making a positive contribution and achieving economic well-being
- *Our Health, Our Care, Our Say* (DoH 2006b) – the key policy document for the provision of integrated services in the community, which refers explicitly to sexual health services

- *Creating a Patient-led NHS: Delivering the NHS Improvement Plan* (DoH 2005a) – which focuses on encouraging informed choice and on NHS organisations becoming more focused and better at understanding the needs of their patients and commissioning services that more effectively meet the needs of the local population.

While a national commitment to improving sexual health in key policy documents is welcomed, it is important that these policies are a real lever for change at the local level, which in turn will lead to improvements in sexual health outcomes for our populations.

Real changes are happening. While England still has one of the highest teenage conception rates in western Europe, UK teenage pregnancy rates are at their lowest for twenty years. Waiting times at GUM clinics have improved from 38% of patients seen within 48 hours in May 2004, to 57% in August 2006. There has been an increase in uptake of HIV testing in GUM clinics among gay and bisexual men from 64% in 2003 to 79% in 2004 and in heterosexuals, an increase in testing uptake from 54% in 2003 to at least 75% in 2004 (DoH 2006b).

Many areas now have chlamydia screening programmes in place and, if not, are well on their way to having opportunistic screening programmes for all under-25-year-old men and women in the community by April 2007. The National Chlamydia Screening Programme was set up following the recommendations in *Choosing Health*. This service has a community focus and concentrates on opportunistic screening of asymptomatic sexually active men and women under age of 25 who would not normally access, or be offered a chlamydia test, and focuses on screening in non-traditional sites (youth services, military bases, universities, contraception services, primary care) (DoH 2005b).

While there are real improvements being made in improving sexual health and sexual health services, a long-term commitment is required if we are to really improve sexual health and more importantly ensure that these improvements are sustainable.

A major modernisation of the whole range of NHS sexual health services is needed with emphasis on offering more locally based, accessible services for testing and screening for STIs and targeting young people, vulnerable people and those who are hard to reach or at significant risk, such as black and minority ethnic groups.

We hope that *Choosing Health* will drive the modernisation of sexual health services. So far, £130 million has been promised to modernise GUM clinics, with an additional £80 million to complete the national rollout of the chlamydia screening programme.

There is also a commitment to spending £50 million on a sexual health advertising campaign for under-25s and further financial support to upgrade prevention services including contraceptive services.

If this strategy is adequately supported, it will go some way to halting the worryingly high levels of poor sexual health; but the financial and political commitment by the government and the commitment to implement at the local level must be real. Already some PCTs are being accused of not allocating *Choosing Health* monies towards improvements in sexual health and instead are using the monies to maintain financial balance at year-end. A recent report in Public Health News (2006) reported that 64 GUM providers have had difficulty in getting any of their *Choosing Health* funds allocated to develop services and in other areas, plans to develop chlamydia screening programmes have been halted.

The role of the midwife

As midwives we should be moving away from a medical model that tends to diagnose and treat and tends to be service-centred, which can fragment care. We should be working towards a social model of health that encourages a holistic approach encompassing the wider determinants of health. These models are discussed in Chapter 1. Pregnancy presents an ideal window of opportunity for many issues, especially for promoting sexual health, and midwives need to be able to offer signposting, advice and support in a non-judgmental way. Advice for subsequent pregnancies and contraception can include a sexual health check, especially around screening, safe sex and access to information around treatment.

In 2006, the policy document *Teenage Pregnancy: Accelerating the Strategy to 2010* (DfES 2006) was issued. This document aims to assist local areas in meeting their 2010 target of halving teenage conceptions. The document highlights examples of best practice from across the country and makes recommendations for implementation that will make a real difference to meeting the target. In relation to preventing repeat pregnancies, it specifically refers to the role of the midwife as follows:

We have made clear in the Childrens Centres Practice Guidance and Maternity standard of the National Service Framework, the critical importance of supporting teenage parents to access a method of contraception they are confident to use. We will also be liaising with relevant professional bodies for midwives and health visitors, including the Royal Colleges, to build contraception training into preregistration and CPD programmes

(DfES 2006)

In October 2005, NICE published guidance on long-acting reversible contraception (LARC). The guidance aims to assist clinicians and patients in making decisions about the most appropriate treatment for specific conditions.

LARC is taken up by an estimated 8% of women aged 16–49 years (2003–2004). Oral contraceptives and male condoms are the most commonly used methods of contraception, with uptake of 25% and 23% respectively. Uptake of LARC is fairly low when compared with other contraceptive methods (NICE 2005).

It is vital that midwives are up-to-date with recommendations such as those in the NICE guidance. Midwives are well placed to discuss future contraceptive use. The option of using LARC may be of particular benefit to women who have more difficulty in complying with a contraceptive that needs to be taken on a daily basis, e.g. the pill, and also for those women who may have a particularly erratic lifestyle. However, the guidelines do highlight that – particularly for young women and those who are considered to be at greater risk of infection – health professionals need to stress that LARC does not provide protection against sexually transmitted infections and that barrier methods, e.g. the condom should still be used in addition to LARC.

NICE has also recently produced draft guidance on public health interventions in relation to sexual health and these were out for consultation at the time of writing (NICE 2006). The draft guidance is entitled *One-to-one interventions to reduce the transmission of sexually transmitted infections (STIs) including HIV, and to reduce the rate of under-18 conceptions, especially among vulnerable and at-risk groups.*

Recommendation 6 explicitly refers to midwifery. It states that those who provide antenatal, postnatal and child development services should regularly visit vulnerable women, aged 18 and under, who are pregnant or already mothers and discuss and provide information about preventing sexually transmitted infections and LARC in line with the NICE clinical guideline.

Pregnancy does not protect against sexually transmitted infections and yet some women will continue to practice high-risk sexual behaviours in pregnancy. Condoms are often seen as contraceptive rather than preventive, but the protective elements of condoms should be discussed sensitively with pregnant women.

Research by Dwyer (2001) found that pregnant women were largely unaware about the dangers associated with sexually transmitted infections during pregnancy. She found that 91% of couples rarely or never used condoms, either before or during pregnancy, despite the fact that 95% of women were unaware of their partner's infection status. More than half of the women sampled were ignorant about the effect of sexually transmitted infections on their pregnancy. More than one-quarter of the women (27%) had multiple partners during their pregnancy.

We have already discussed the National Chlamydia Screening Programme and how the programme offers opportunistic screening to under-25s in community settings and aims to pick up those asymptomatic young people and their partners who otherwise would not have come forward for testing. There has been some discussion nationally around whether or not chlamydia screening for the under-25s should become a standard screen offered to pregnant women as chlamydia infection can be transmitted from mother to child. Screening may be an effective mechanism for reducing this transmission as some treatments for chlamydia can be prescribed during pregnancy.

However, Sir Muir Gray, Programme Director of the UK National Screening Committee issued a letter to the National Chlamydia Screening Programme highlighting the Committee's current policy on chlamydia screening. Where chlamydia screening is already being carried out in antenatal clinics it can continue; but where screening is not being offered in pregnancy it should not be added to the range of tests offered to a woman until that programme has met its screening target for Down's syndrome, cystic fibrosis, sickle cell anaemia and thalassaemia and has all midwives trained in the physical examination of the newborn (UK National Screening Committee 2006). So while chlamydia screening for all pregnant women is not being offered at the moment, it may be an option for consideration in the future.

There may be many reasons why midwives do not discuss safer sex during pregnancy. It may be that midwives are unsure of their own knowledge base around sexual health or are anxious about upsetting women or their partners. Or they may be embarrassed about discussing sexual health issues. However, the fact that women are pregnant means that they have had unprotected sex and although this does mean they have had unsafe sex, there are ideal opportunities to deliver sexual health promotion messages during pregnancy. Key times for discussion include booking, screening visits, if the midwife is aware of a change of partner and during the postnatal period.

Information and useful resources

Sexual health is everybody's business and midwives can have an influential role in improving the sexual health of our population. These resources provide further information and guidance for those of you who may be interested in developing your knowledge and skills around this area of work.

Department of Health

www.dh.gov.uk

- Better prevention, better services, better sexual health: The national strategy for sexual health and HIV
- Best practice guidance for doctors and other health professionals on the provision of advice and treatment to young people under 16 on contraception, sexual and reproductive health
- Effective sexual health promotion toolkit: a toolkit for primary care trusts and others working in the field of promoting good sexual health and HIV prevention
- A competency framework for nurses working in the specialty of sexual and reproductive health across the United Kingdom
- *Recommended quality standards for sexual health training* – good practice guidance on the provision of sexual health training
- *Recommended standards for sexual health services* – this document is intended for those involved in planning, commissioning and providing sexual health services. It provides a comprehensive set of recommended service standards, with supporting evidence.

Teenage Pregnancy Unit

www.teenagepregnancyunit.gov.uk
Information about:

- National strategy
- Latest data on conception rates
- Guidance issued by the Teenage Pregnancy Unit
- Examples of promising practice
- Research reports
- Relevant publications from other government departments

- Implementation of local strategy
- The Independent Advisory Group on Teenage Pregnancy.

British Association for Sexual Health and HIV (BASHH)

www.bashh.org
   BASHH aims to:

- Promote, encourage and improve the study and practice of diagnosing and treating STIs
- Promote and encourage the study of the public aspects of STIs
- Educate the public about GUM
- Promote a high standard in GUM.

Family Planning Association

www.fpa.org.uk
   The fpa is a charity working to improve the sexual health of all people throughout the UK. They work with the public and professionals to ensure that high quality information and services are available to everyone who needs them. The website contains:

- Advice for women who think they may be pregnant, or who have had unprotected sex
- Sex statistics and facts
- A comprehensive guide to all methods of contraception.

Health Protection Agency

www.hpa.org.uk
   The Health Protection Agency provides epidemiological data on HIV and AIDS and other sexually transmitted infections.

Medical Foundation for AIDS and Sexual Health (Medfash)

www.medfash.org.uk
   The Medical Foundation for AIDS and Sexual Health is a charity which works with policy-makers and health professionals, to promote excellence in the prevention and management of HIV and other sexually transmitted infections.

National AIDS Trust (NAT)

www.nat.org.uk

The National AIDS Trust (NAT) is the UK's leading independent policy and campaigning voice on HIV and AIDS. It develops policies and campaigns to halt the spread of HIV and AIDS, and improve the quality of life of people affected by HIV, both in the UK and internationally. It aims to:

- Prevent the spread of HIV and AIDS
- Ensure people living with HIV have access to treatment and care
- Eradicate HIV-related stigma and discrimination.

Key implications for midwifery practice

- Engage with your PCT and School Health service to offer support and advice to young people.
- Encourage condom use for women with a new or casual partner.
- Advise women to have a check up if they have put themselves at risk of acquiring a STI or have any symptoms.
- Pregnancy and the postnatal period are windows of opportunity to influence future sexual health.
- Do you know where your local GUM clinic is? What advice and treatment is offered?
- Is there a Brook clinic or another young person's sexual health service in your area? Do you know how to refer young women?
- Who is your local teenage pregnancy co-ordinator?
- Is there a chlamydia screening programme offered in your area?
- Do you have access to condom distribution?
- Are there opportunities for midwives to access additional training around family planning and sexual health?

References

Armstrong N, Davey C, Donaldson C (2005) *The Economics of Sexual Health: Findings*. London, fpa.

Blacksmith E (2000) *Sex in the Middle Ages*. www.rencentral.com/feb_mar_vol2/sexmiddleages.shtml (accessed 5/12/2006).

Botting B, Rosato M, Wood R (1998) Teenage mothers and the health of their children. *Population Trends* 93, Autumn.

Dawe F, Meltzer M (1999) *Contraception and Sexual Health 1999*: A report on using the ONS Omnibus survey produced on behalf of the Department of Health. London, National Statistics.

Department for Education and Skills (2004) *Every Child Matters: Change for Children.* London, The Stationery Office. www.dfes.gov.uk/everychildmatters/ (accessed 4/12/06).

Department for Education and Skills (2006) *Teenage Pregnancy: Accelerating the Strategy to 2010.* London, DfES.

Department of Health (1999) *Teenage Pregnancy: a Social Exclusion Unit Report.* London, DoH.

Department of Health (2000) *Trends in sexually transmitted infections in the United Kingdom, 1990–1999. New episodes seen at genitourinary medicine clinics:* PHLS (England, Wales and Northern Ireland), DHSS and PS (Northern Ireland).

Department of Health (2001) *The National Strategy for Sexual Health and HIV.* London, DoH.

Department of Health (2002) *The National Strategy For Sexual Health And HIV Action Plan.* London, DoH.

Department of Health (2004a) *Choosing Health White Paper.* London, DoH.

Department of Health (2004b) Independent Advisory Group on Sexual Health and HIV: Response to the Health Select Committee Report on Sexual Health. London, DoH.

Department of Health (2005a) *Creating a Patient-led NHS: Delivering the NHS Improvement Plan.* www.dh.gov.uk/PublicationsAndStatistics/Publications/PublicationsPolicyAndGuidance/PublicationsPolicyAndGuidanceArticle/fs/en?CONTENT_ID=4106506&chk=ftV6vA (accessed 5/12/06).

Department of Health (2005b) *National Chlamydia Screening Programme: Phase 3 Guide.* London, DoH.

Department of Health (2006a) *Fact Sheet on Sexual Health.* London, DoH.

Department of Health (2006b) *Our Health, Our Care, Our Say: a New Direction for Community Services.* London, The Stationery Office. www.dh.gov.uk/PublicationsAndStatistics/Publications/PublicationsPolicyAndGuidance/fs/en (accessed 4/12/06).

Dwyer JM (2001) High-risk sexual behaviours and genital infections during pregnancy. *International Nurse Reviewer* 48(4): 233–40.

Ellis S, Barnett-Page E, Morgan A (2003) *HIV Prevention:* a review of reviews assessing the effectiveness of interventions to reduce the risk of sexual transmission. London, Health Development Agency.

Erens B, McManus S, Prescott P *et al.* (2003) *National Survey of Sexual Attitudes and Lifestyles II: (NATSAL) reference tables and summary report.* London: National Centre for Social Research.

Fenton KA, Hughes G (2003) Sexual behaviour in Britain: why sexually transmitted infections are common. *Clinical Medicine* 3(3): 199–202.

Health Education Authority (1999) *Young People and Health.* London, HEA.

Health Protection Agency (2001) National Strategy for sexual health and HIV. *CDR Weekly* 31, 2 August 2001, PHLS CDSC. www.hpa.org.uk/cdr/archives/2001/cdr3101.pdf (accessed 13/12/06).

Health Protection Agency (2004) *Focus on Prevention: HIV and other Sexually Transmitted Infections in the United Kingdom in 2003 – an update.* London, HPA.

Health Protection Agency (2005) *HIV and other Sexually Transmitted Infections in the UK.* London, HPA.

Hughes G, Catchpole M, Rogers PA (2000) Comparison of risk factors for sexually transmitted infections: results from a study of attenders at three genitourinary medicine clinics in England. *Sexually Transmitted Infections* 76: 262–67.

Johnson AM, Mercer CH, Erens B *et al.* (2001) Sexual behaviour in Britain: partnerships, practices, and HIV risk behaviours. *Lancet* 358(9296): 1835–42.

Kidd, M-C (2006) NHS cuts hit sexual health services. *Public Health News* 29 October 2006.

National AIDS Trust (2006) www.nat.org.uk/HIV_Facts (accessed 5/12/06).

National AIDS Trust (2006) Public lack of knowledge of HIV. *The Pharmaceutical Journal* 276: 559.

National Chlamydia Screening Steering Group (2005) *Looking Back, Moving Forward.* Annual report of the National Chlamydia Screening Programme (NCSP) in England, 2004/05. London, DoH.

National Institute for Health and Clinical Excellence (2005) *Long-acting Reversible Contraception: The Effective and Appropriate Use of Long-Acting Reversible Contraception, Guideline 30.* October 2005. www.nice.org.uk/275466 (accessed 13/12/06).

National Institute for Health and Clinical Excellence (2006) *Preventing Sexually Transmitted Infections and Reducing Under-18 Conceptions* (draft guidance for consultation). www.nice.org.uk/page.aspx?o=371780 (accessed 5/12/06).

Office of National Statistics (2004) Teenage conceptions: by age at conception and outcome, 2001. *Social Trends* 34.

Office for National Statistics (2005) *Under-18 conceptions data for top-tier local authorities* (LAD1), 1998–2003. Version 24.02.05. Office for National Statistics and the Teenage Pregnancy Unit.

Ridgway S (1997) *Sexuality and Modernity.* www.isis.aust.com/stephan/writings/sexuality/pref.htm (accessed 5/12/06).

Royal College of Obstetricians and Gynaecologists (2005) *National Study of HIV in Pregnancy and Childhood.* www.rcog.org.uk/index.asp?PageID=1422 (accessed 13/12/06).

Rutherford J, Holman R, MacDonald J *et al.* (2006) Low literacy: a hidden problem in family planning clinics. *Journal of Family Planning and Reproductive Health Care* 32(4): 235–240.

Sefton AM (2001) The Great Pox that was syphilis. *Journal of Applied Microbiology* 91: 592–96.

Simms I, Stephenson JM (2000) Pelvic inflammatory disease epidemiology: what do we know and what do we need to know? *Sexually Transmitted Infections* 76: 80–87.

Social Exclusion Unit (1999) *Teenage Pregnancy*. London, The Stationery Office.

UK National Screening Committee. Letter from Sir Muir Gray, 22 March 2006. www.nsc.nhs.uk/uk_nsc/meeting150305.pdf (accessed 13/12/06).

World Health Organization (2006) *Sexual Health*. www.who.int/reproductive-health/gender/sexual_health.html#3 (accessed 5/12/06).

Chapter 6
Substance Misuse: What is the Problem?

Lyn McIver

> Treatment for substance abuse during pregnancy can be more
> effective than at other times in a woman's life
>
> (DoH 2000)

Social context

Substance misuse may involve many different substances including smoking, alcohol and drugs, and a body of evidence exists that
all three have a detrimental effect on health. During the childbirth
period, however, the potential for harm is doubled as negative
consequences may involve the baby and the mother.

Smoking as a public health issue was discussed in detail in
Chapter 3. This chapter will concentrate on illegal drug and alcohol misuse, and the consequences for the mother and her baby.

The vision of the NHS Plan (DoH 1999) was to set out a long-
term strategy for reform and improvements in the UK. The document detailed a new way of delivering care and highlighted the
importance of the patient as being central to determining their
own needs and in influencing health and social care systems. For
maternity services, the Plan reflected the underpinning philosophy of *Changing Childbirth* (1993), and is affirmed in the *National
Service Framework for Children, Young People and Maternity Services*
(DoH 2004a) in the promotion of woman-centred care; a fundamental element when planning or delivering care for women who
misuse substances during the childbirth continuum.

Although drug use occurs across the spectrum of all social
classes there is a recognised associated link with social deprivation. Over the past 50 years there has been a shift in the type of
drugs and the age of those who use drugs.

Changing demographics of drug misuse

The first legislation on drugs of dependence in the UK was followed by the Dangerous Drugs Act 1920, which allowed doctors to use narcotic drugs as a form of medical treatment. The Rolleston Report published in 1926 formed the first defined policy on the treatment of drug dependence in the UK, providing flexibility for clinicians and included advice on:

- Gradual withdrawal of a drug
- If attempts to withdraw have failed, then maintenance can be achieved to enable a person to lead what is regarded as a normal life as possible with opportunities to move from the current situation to a more productive one that reduces the level of drug misuse or achieves abstinence.

This principle of maintenance became known as the 'British System' of treatment and care.

In the 1960s individuals who misused drugs were typically middle-aged and did so for recreation. But there was a shift in the late 1960s with the emergence of young opiate drug users. The Brain Report (1961) suggested that there was no cause for concern. By 1965 the profile had changed and a second report by Brain (1965) highlighted a new, young, unstable population who used drugs. In response to this report, psychiatric-led secondary drug services were established, commonly referred to as drug dependency clinics, which were often based in densely populated areas. Until then, treatment had been with general practitioners (GPs) in primary care, and concerns about transfer to specialist services were raised in relation to the deskilling of GPs.

With the 1970s came the development of prescribed drugs for addiction, predominantly methadone and a rise in the number of drug users presenting for treatment. Two decades later the numbers of patients presenting continues to rise both in the general population and across the range of treatment services.

In an attempt to monitor this rise in England, the National Drug Treatment Monitoring System (NDTMS) was established. It is currently managed by the National Treatment Agency for Substance Misuse (NTA) and operated by nine regional centres. The NTA monitors the performance of the drug treatment system across England. The regional team collects data from all of the region's structured drug treatment providers. This is then collated by the NTA and monthly figures are produced for each Drug (and Alcohol) Action Team (D(A)AT).

NDTMS figures are used to monitor the government's commitment to double the number of people receiving drug treatment between 1998 and 2008. The same figures are also used as part of the Healthcare Commission's 'star ratings' system for performance managing primary care trusts (PCTs) and mental health trusts. The current number of people in drug treatment services in May 2006 was 140 319 (NTA 2006a), and commissioners base their local drug services on this data.

For the past 20 years, the Department of Health has conducted a large-scale survey of 9000 11–15-year-olds to identify trends in smoking, alcohol and drug taking. In 2005, 19% of respondents had taken drugs in the previous year, a similar proportion to 2004 (18%) and a decrease from 21% in 2003 (DoH 2005).

As in previous years, prevalence of drug taking increased with age: 6% of 11-year-olds had taken drugs in the last year compared with 34% of 15-year-olds. In 2005, as in previous years, young people were more likely to use cannabis than any other drug. Twelve percent of pupils aged 11–15 had used cannabis in the last year, a similar proportion to 2004 (11%). The prevalence in both 2005 and 2004 was lower than in 2003 (13%) (DoH 2005).

Illegal drugs and their effects

It is important for midwives to have a broad understanding of the common illegal recreation drugs used, how they are used and their effects.

Heroin and methadone

The most commonly used and available illicit drug used by women during pregnancy is heroin, bought on the streets or used as part of a partner's prescribed dose. Heroin is short-acting opium with marked withdrawal effects, including muscle spasm. One of the problems of taking heroin or methadone is that the woman may stop having periods. There is an increased risk of miscarriage in the first trimester of pregnancy, when the woman may not have realised that she has conceived and has continued taking drugs. Women may prefer to use their partner's heroin. This enables them to stay out of the drug treatment system that represents, for some women, authority and involvement of social care and child protection system, concluding in a fear that their babies will be removed from them because they are unfit mothers.

Methadone is prescribed as a safer alternative to heroin as it can be administered orally as opposed to injecting, thereby reducing some of the harm-related risks. The use of methadone as a stabilisation and maintenance drug, especially in the first and third trimesters, shows better outcomes.

Stabilisation during pregnancy remains at the centre of the integrated care planning for pregnant women. Women who access services during pregnancy are predominantly prescribed oral methadone as an opiate substitute to enable a stabilisation process to occur. Treatment management should be tailored to the needs of the individual women. Buprenorphine, an opiate antagonist, is increasingly being used as an alternative during pregnancy as an opioid substitute.

Benzodiazepines

The use of diazepam and chlordiazepoxide during the first trimester of pregnancy has been associated with an increased risk of congenital malformations, and fetal damage may be caused by the use of benzodiazepines during pregnancy. Benzodiazepines, as with methadone, have a long half-life and it is necessary to observe the baby for up to two days. It is not known whether such drugs are passed in the breastmilk.

Withdrawal from opiates and benzodiazepines can cause significant problems and there may be a need for a range of treatments from simple measures such as gentle handling and comfort to sedatives, opiates and anticonvulsant therapy. Additional symptoms may be manifested in the babies of poly drug users, e.g. occurrence of convulsions at an earlier stage.

Cocaine

Cocaine readily crosses the placenta and affects the fetus. It constricts blood vessels, possibly reducing blood flow (and the oxygen supply), which may in turn slow the growth of the fetus, particularly of the bones and the intestine. Where babies are affected, they are more likely to be small and to have a small head. Rarely, use of cocaine results in birth defects of the brain, eyes, kidneys, and genital organs.

Use of cocaine during pregnancy can also cause pregnancy complications. Among women who use cocaine throughout pregnancy, there is an increase in preterm delivery and placental abruption.

The chances of a miscarriage are also increased. Low birthweight infants are more common.

Marijuana

Whether use of marijuana during pregnancy can harm the fetus is unclear. The main ingredient of marijuana, tetrahydrocannabinol, can cross the placenta and may affect the fetus. If marijuana is used heavily during pregnancy, the baby may have behavioural problems.

If the woman injects any of the substances listed above, advice should be given to minimise risks and she should be offered support to reduce or preferably stop injecting. Injecting into the veins of the breast, abdomen and femoral areas should be discouraged, as abscesses and deep vein thrombosis can occur. These complications should be assessed at each contact visit with the midwife and care given as appropriate. Partners sometimes take the responsibility for injecting the woman, and may continue to do this in the hospital setting. These issues should be discussed sensitively with the couple in a non-judgmental manner.

Women with problematic substance misuse are considered high risk during pregnancy, and need to be informed of the potential effects on the child. Drugs taken in pregnancy reach the fetus primarily by crossing the placenta, the same route taken by oxygen and nutrients, which are needed for growth and development. The drugs may affect the fetus in several ways:

- Act directly on the fetus, causing damage, abnormal development (leading to birth defects), or death
- Alter the function of the placenta, usually by constricting blood vessels and reducing the supply of oxygen and nutrients to the fetus from the mother and thus sometimes resulting in a baby that is growth-retarded
- Cause the muscles of the uterus to contract forcefully, indirectly injuring the fetus by reducing its blood supply or triggering preterm labour and delivery
- Initiate a range of symptoms in the neonatal period known as neonatal abstinence syndrome along a spectrum ranging from sneezing, poor feeding, tremors to restlessness. Symptoms are reported to occur more generally from the age of 48 hours and may last for week or months. (Shaw and McIvor 1995).

The infant may also have been put at risk of the transmission of blood-borne viruses, e.g. HIV, herpes and hepatitis B and C.

Alcohol

Pregnant women should be advised to keep to the guidelines of no more than one or two units once or twice a week, which includes both the level and pattern of consumption (MIDIRS 2005). Several risk factors emerge for women who consume large amounts in pregnancy. Fetal alcohol effects (FAE) is a term used to describe the many problems associated with exposure to alcohol before birth. The most severe of these is fetal alcohol syndrome (FAS), a combination of physical and mental birth defects. Fetal alcohol syndrome is a common cause of mental retardation and is characterised by a set of features in a neonate. The features of FAS include pre and postnatal growth retardation, mental retardation/learning disabilities and facial abnormalities including flattened midface, sunken nasal bridge, flattened and elongated philtrum (groove between nose and lips) and various degrees of organ malformations.

As the children grow, they may demonstrate learning difficulties and neurodevelopmental disorder. This syndrome is associated with children of women who chronically misuse alcohol or indulge in 'binge drinking' rather than social drinkers, but this is not always the case. At all points along the continuum from occasional light drinking to regular heavy drinking there is conflicting evidence as to the possibility of damaging effects on the fetus (Mounteney 1999). According to Abel and Sokol (1991), FAS occurs among the general population of the Western world at the rate of one per 3000 live births. Estimates have placed FAE at about three per 3000 live births. However, a conservative estimate – nearly one in every 100 live births – confirms the perception of many health professionals that fetal alcohol exposure is a serious problem.

The burden of alcohol-related illness on the NHS has been debated by the Royal College of Physicians (2001). As with illicit drugs, alcohol use crosses all social boundaries, with the associated consequences of comorbidity, family and relationship breakdown, crime and unemployment. This has the potential to have a devastating effect on future generations.

Current drug service provision

In 2003 the Drug Intervention Programme was introduced as a critical part of the government's strategy for tackling drugs. The programme aimed to develop and integrate interventions to help adult offenders who misuse drugs out of crime and into treatment (see www.drugs.uk).

The programme provides this client group (which includes women) convicted of crime and entering the criminal justice system with opportunities to undergo a range of treatment services instead of receiving custodial sentences. This alternative route is especially important for pregnant drug users, as it is known that prison can have detrimental effects on both the woman and her baby. Problems may include separation, rejection, mental health problems and feeling of guilt by the mother.

Currently, the UK national strategy is aimed at enabling illicit drug users to access treatment services appropriate to their need and keep drug users engaged for a minimum of 12 weeks. These targets provide access into a range of services that complement hospital and community-based midwifery services. A wide range of services exist in local settings, often working in partnership to enable an individual to move from one service to another dependent on their need and the appropriateness of services.

These services are categorised in a tier system:

Tier 1   Services not specific to substance misuse, e.g. one-stop shops, Citizen's Advice Bureau

Tier 2   Open access drug- and alcohol-specific services e.g. counselling services, family support

Tier 3   Structured community-based drug treatment services e.g. community drug teams

Tier 4a Residential drug and alcohol misuse-specific services, e.g. inpatient detoxification

Tier 4b Highly specialist services not specific to substance misuse, e.g. accommodation

This structure aims to enable stability and continuity of treatment options and opportunities for rehabilitation and life-changing circumstances. Ideally any person who uses substances should have equal access to a range of high-quality interventions within treatment services. Several major national and international UK and US drug treatment outcome studies (Simpson and Sells 1983; Hubbard *et al.* 1997; Gossop *et al.* 2003) reported that:

- Substantial reductions in illegal drug misuse and other outcomes were found after treatment.
- Improved outcomes were also found for injecting risk behaviours.

- Most drug dependent clients were multiple substance misusers and often had multiple dependencies and that to focus on one single substance disorder is outdated and misleading.
- Overdose remained a serious problem among drug users with an increased risk of mortality.
- The timing of treatment and completion of treatment programmes was found to be associated with better treatment outcomes.
- The reductions in crime levels provide substantial and immediate cost savings for society.
- Methadone programmes achieved a range of improved client outcomes.
- Case mix differences were found with more severely problematic drug misusers receiving treatment in residential treatment programmes.
- Most drug-dependent clients received more than one episode of treatment.
- Drinking outcomes were often poor, with many clients continuing to drink heavily.
- Treatment of drinking problems should be strengthened.

Many drug services prioritise entry into their service for pregnant women and often her partner, which increases the potential of creating a supportive environment for the couple. Detoxification can be undertaken under supervision at any time and built into a care pathway for individuals. Co-ordination may be necessary to enable support from the partner and to arrange childcare.

Women, vulnerability and drug misuse

There are well-documented adverse effects of substance misuse in pregnancy, making it a vulnerable time for the woman and her unborn child. Hepburn (2005) reported an increased incidence of preterm delivery and low birthweight and an increase in sudden infant deaths in pregnant drug users. Substance misuse during pregnancy adversely affects outcomes both medically and socially.

Some women presenting with drug and alcohol problems may be doubly vulnerable as they may be already marginalised through poverty or have a disadvantaged background. This may include lack of education and employment resulting in low levels of literacy and numeracy. There is often chaos in their lives and complexity in their needs.

Women may be faced with funding a drug habit that is costly and time consuming. Even when pregnant, women could become victims of sexual exploitation to fund their habit, which puts them at risk of blood-borne viruses, drug-related death, physical and psychological danger, degradation and potential death.

Mental health problems are more pronounced in women who misuse drugs (Klee 1997). The Confidential Enquiry into Maternal Deaths in the UK (2002) found disproportionate numbers of deaths in disadvantaged groups. Eight percent of women who died misused substances. Women living in families where both partners were unemployed, many of whom had features of social exclusion, were up to 20 times more likely to die than women from the more advantaged groups (CEMACH 2004).

What can midwives and maternity services do?

For some women, entering a formalised service such as a drug dependency service can be traumatic. Often there is a fear of being judged as being a bad woman and an unfit mother. This may also affect the woman's perception of maternity services, so women who misuse drugs will often present late during pregnancy.

In 1996 the Department of Health released a report of an Independent Review of Drug Treatment Services in England, which highlighted that maternity staff felt ill equipped to work with pregnant women who misuse drugs. This led to the introduction of specialist midwives, a role that aims to provide easier access to all services, continuity of care and contact on a regular basis. The specialist post facilitates direct access to maternity services and provides opportunities for the midwife to:

- take the lead
- liaise with other agencies
- provide continuity of care
- act as the woman's advocate
- develop expertise in drug dependency, blood-borne viruses and aspects of addiction, through education and training in maternity services and across agencies.

All midwives need to be aware of the special needs of vulnerable women. For the woman, pregnancy can act as a strong incentive to make a positive change to substance-misusing behaviour. This presents the midwife with a window of opportunity to enquire sensitively about any substance use and to provide necessary support and signposting to relevant agencies to reduce harm. Siney (2005), outlines the evolving role of the midwife in recent years in a public health framework, developing an understanding of the common risks associated with drug use and/or alcohol dependency and what they are able to offer in the way of support.

If possible, a named midwife or specialist midwife should liaise with the range of services involved and co-ordinate care

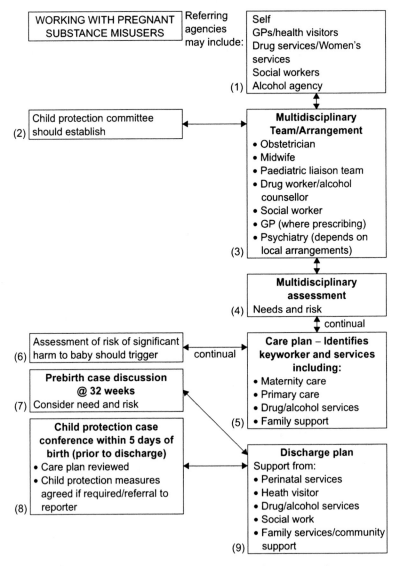

Figure 6.1 Example of an integrated care pathway for pregnant drug users.
Source: Scottish Executive (2006).

throughout the pregnancy. This will include care from a multidisciplinary team, who will facilitate streamlined care provision for the health and social needs of both mother and baby. The main focus of care should be to reduce harm by facilitating the stabilisation on prescribed medication. It is important to remember that some women also have a fear that prescribed methadone will lead to increased symptoms and may choose to continue using street drugs.

In 2004 the Department of Health (2004a) set standards for maternity services to be proactive in engaging all women, but especially those from vulnerable groups. The document also encouraged the development of specialist services for complex care, including women who misuse drugs.

Scotland has developed effective responses to caring for pregnant women who misuse drugs. The UK Scottish Executive recognises that:

> A new approach is needed to address risks and needs. As a first step this should start with assessing the needs of all newborn babies born to drug or alcohol misusing parents
>
> (Scottish Executive 2001)

Models of care

The UK government introduced the Models of Care (NTA 2002) document to complement the existing national service frameworks. Models of Care aims to standardise levels of care in the formation of integrated care pathways and processes nationally. It functions in a similar way to national service frameworks in recognising the complex needs of individuals and the multiagency approach to the delivery of care. Models of care should be taken in the context of the maternity service framework and other associated policies to achieve consistency and avoid duplication.

Local drug and alcohol action teams (strategic partnerships) were challenged with the introduction and implementation of the Models of Care within their strategic plans and annual treatment plans. National guidelines have been produced on the management of substance misuse in pregnancy and should be reflected on to service policies. Midwifery and neonatal staff will need training to inform them of the process and to involve them in the consultation and implementation periods.

Service user consultation – both locally and nationally – enables the Models of Care process to use patients' experience and to document their journeys in both drug and maternity services. Users of substance-misusing services should be integral to service structures. Involving them in, for example, maternity service liaison committees enables them to review, contribute to service and policy development and have a direct impact on patient care.

The newly introduced Healthcare Commission reviews NHS investments and develops health improvement plans where necessary. To support the continued work and governance of services, specialists in the field review both statutory and voluntary services. In relation to substance misuse services, they will assess the management, provision and quality of NHS healthcare and public health services and monitor complaints. All trusts will be measured by an annual health check and will be expected to show evidence of real progress in meeting nationally agreed standards of care. In carrying out the duties of the Healthcare Commission, trusts are required to pay particular attention to the availability of, access to, quality and effectiveness of healthcare, including substance misuse services and will provide a useful benchmark for ensuring the quality of services we offer. For more information on the work of the Healthcare Commission, visit www.healthcarecommission.org.uk.

In 2006 there was an update to the Models of Care to reflect the recommendations of the government monitoring system *Standards for Better Health* (NTA 2006b; DoH 2004b). The guidelines, which are based on the best available evidence, support woman-centred care, particularly for vulnerable women, and will help women receive effective treatment and care that conforms to nationally agreed best practice, particularly as defined in the agreed national guidance on service delivery. The new Model strongly supports a seamless service across all organisations that need to be involved, especially social care organisations.

By adopting a public health–social model of care in the delivery of maternity services, healthcare workers can contribute to maximising health and social outcomes for future generations. Public health practitioners, treatment services and midwifery staff all have responsibility to provide accessible, appropriate services to this client group, and commissioners are key to the process. As mentioned previously, the collation and analysis of drug misuse data has been devolved to commissioners, and it may also be used to inform and influence associated funding streams and local delivery plans across health and social care.

Additional concepts of treatment include assessment of need in regard to housing, social and education and employment needs. Joint assessment clinics which aim at providing a multiagency approach to the care of pregnant drug users create opportunities for proactive and preventive work to be undertaken, and for parenting skills to be developed.

Women should be actively encouraged to participate in the planning of their care at each stage. The midwife and all health and social care workers should strive to work alongside the woman, caring for her in a non-judgmental way. Information should be given objectively and sensitively on how her baby may be treated for symptoms and she should be encouraged and supported to care for her baby, if possible from birth. This is aided by arrangements that support transitional care in the postnatal period so that the woman and her baby are not separated. Pre-birth meetings with the woman and her family during the antenatal period can help to relieve some of the anxieties that women may experience. These meetings must be informal, non-judgmental and informative. Support would be the main purpose of the session, and the woman should be given every opportunity to participate in any decisions made about her and her baby's care.

Breastfeeding

Mothers who misuse substances and who are prescribed methadone should be encouraged to breastfeed as other mothers, providing their drug use is stable and the baby is weaned gradually. Successful establishment of breastfeeding is in itself a marker of adequate stability of drug use (Drug Misuse in Pregnancy Breastfeeding Project (2003)). However, breastfeeding should not be encouraged, if a woman is:

- Using multiple substances in large quantities
- Using in a very inconsistent manner
- Injecting drugs
- Using cocaine, crack or large doses of amphetamines
- HIV-positive (Day and George 2005)

To enable effective breastfeeding and the development of appropriate attachment, babies should be cared for by their parents wherever possible. Unnecessarily prolonged hospitalisation or placement away from the parents should be avoided. Withdrawal symptoms at birth in a baby subject to fetal addiction may make the baby more difficult to care for in the postnatal period. If the baby experiences withdrawal symptoms or has other health problems, maternity services should provide full information about the child's care, progress and any prognosis to the parent(s) with sensitivity.

Drug misuse and child protection

A major form of stress and concern expressed by women is the fear of the baby experiencing withdrawal from the effects of their drug use. This may mean a woman does not disclose her drug status until the baby starts to withdraw after delivery. Experienced staff may identify a baby displaying signs of withdrawal and sensitive discussion with the mother may encourage the women to disclose substance misuse. Different substances are known to have different effects on the behaviour that may, in turn, impact on childcare such as neglect, risk of injury and poor parenting (Drummond and Fitzpatrick 2000). Although substance misuse does not necessarily lead to problems in childcare or the neglect or abuse of children it can affect the welfare of children. The Home Office report *Hidden Harm* (2003) provided a grim overview on the effect of parental drug taking on children. The key findings of the research were:

- There are between 250 000 and 350 000 children of problem drug users in the UK – about one for every problem drug user.
- Parental problem drug use can and does cause serious harm to children at every age from conception to adulthood.
- Reducing the harm to children from parental problem drug use should become a main objective of policy and practice.
- Effective treatment of the parent can have major benefits for the child.
- By working together, services can take many practical steps to protect and improve the health and well-being of affected children.
- The number of affected children is only likely to decrease when the number of problem drug users decreases.

(The Home Office 2003)

Pre-birth meetings and working proactively with the woman and her family and relevant organisations – such as the NSPCC or Children's Society – may help to facilitate preventive interventions. This includes one-to-one support and counselling in parenting skills. The role of Children's Centres in providing targeted, locally accessible support is discussed on pages 38. Hepburn (1999) reviewed the social factors that contribute to drug use in pregnancy, and the role of collaboration between agencies and services in providing solutions to the problem.

Should child protection issues be a factor, a planning co-ordination meeting should be convened followed by a structured case conference in partnership with the social services department to consider all factors. The woman, her family and significant others in her family network should be central to all decision making. Communication is essential at all times to ensure an open and transparent process. Case conferences may seem extremely daunting and threatening for any individuals, in particular those who may be using illicit drugs, are in treatment and may also have a history of crime.

Work by Kennel and Klaus (1998) has for the last three decades described the importance of the bond between parents and their infants in the hope that an understanding of relationships would result in improved perinatal care and a reduction in problems such as child abuse, neglect and failure to thrive.

Blood-borne viruses

A major risk of substance misuse, particularly if drugs are injected, is the risk of contracting blood-borne viruses, predominantly hepatitis B and C and, in some cases, HIV. Antenatal screening is of the utmost importance with referral for positive results to infectious disease services. Counselling and support are provided by trained personnel to provide the optimum care and reduce risks where possible. If women are not immune to hepatitis B, a course of vaccine should be offered postnatally. If the mother is hepatitis antigen-positive the baby should be offered active immunisation at birth and passive immunisation by the administration of immunoglobulin with the mother's consent. Information and advice should be provided in written, verbal and media forms and reaffirmed throughout the pregnancy and should be available in various languages and Braille to meet the needs of diverse groups.

Hepatitis C is rapidly emerging as a public health threat to drug users and to the general population as a whole. The British Liver Trust (2005) estimates there are currently 4500 people living with severe liver disease as a result of having a chronic hepatitis C infection and forecasts that the figure could rise to around 7000 by the year 2010. Hepatitis C, sometimes referred to as Hep C or HCV, is a liver disease caused by the hepatitis C virus. The commonest cause is infection with a virus, but inflammation can be caused by excessive alcohol intake, side effects of some drugs and chemicals, and a liver disease, autoimmune hepatitis, in which the body's immune system malfunctions and affects the liver. Other viruses that affect the liver are hepatitis A, B, D and E. The main difference between the viruses is their transmission mode, the effect on the liver and the effect on health in general.

Hepatitis C is transmitted through:

Contact with blood   This may be through sexual intercourse or because of other reasons, for example, sharing a personal item such as a toothbrush or razor.

Sexual activity   There is some evidence that those with many sexual partners and not using a barrier method of contraception have an increased risk of being infected.

Injecting drug use   Current evidence suggests that 50–80% of past and present users may be infected with hepatitis C. They become infected by sharing any equipment used to inject, because it is likely to have invisible contamination with blood. There has been recent concern about sharing straws for snorting cocaine, as the practice may result in infection through nosebleeds (Harsch *et al.* 2000).

Mother-to-baby transmission

The risk of a mother with hepatitis C infecting her baby during pregnancy or during the birth is approximately 6%, but ascertaining time of infection is difficult. It does not occur during conception but is transmitted vertically (Ohto *et al.* 1994).

Babies are sometimes found to have antibodies to the virus, but these usually disappear by the time the baby is 12 to 18 months old, demonstrating that antibodies are passed from mother to baby. Diagnosis may not be possible until the baby is more than one year old, but there is a polymerase chain reaction (PCR) test that may detect the virus in the first few months.

Women who are hepatitis-positive require focused counselling and sensitive support to reduce the stress that may be experienced with concern for potential effects on the fetus. Media information campaigns are increasing understanding of hepatitis – this will increase public awareness and access to screening and testing. Infected mothers are often concerned about passing the virus on to their other children, but the risk of transmission is low and parents can be reassured that kissing and cuddling a child is safe.

Pregnant women who use drugs and who have been involved in high-risk behaviours may present as HIV-positive. The risk is of vertical transmission of infection to the fetus, occurring at any time of pregnancy but in particular at the time of delivery. All women should be given information to enable them to make an informed choice about testing, treatment and obstetric management.

Conclusion

The pregnant woman who uses drugs may present challenges and concerns for those providing care. Listening to the woman and her family is of paramount importance, throughout the whole childbirth continuum and beyond. Often, due to the nature of the women's addiction, the environment in which they find themselves leads to resistance, reluctance to seek support and fear of authority. Midwives and all healthcare workers who come into contact with women who misuse substances must consider each woman as an individual. Maternity services should promote a culture of non-judgmental care to all women, including those who misuse substances (Drummond and Fitzpatrick 2000).

For midwives, careful early assessment of women who misuse drugs, alcohol or substances provides an opportunity for referral to appropriate services. This may be facilitated by a nominated drug liaison midwife or any midwife in maternity services. Education plays a major role in the development of midwifery roles and the delivery of services. Joint training opportunities enable a common vision of maternity and drug treatment care for this client group.

The role of the midwife is central to the health and well-being of all pregnant women, especially those women who are vulnerable, as described in Chapter 1. The midwife is in a position to provide information on health issues, assessment, review, support and specific care during the pregnancy, birth and after delivery. Maternity services offer an opportunity to be involved in wider partnership working and developing new roles through joint working and placements with a range of organisations that include community drug services.

Key implications for midwifery practice

- Think about how you speak to and care for women who misuse substances, and remember their double vulnerability.
- How many pregnant women misuse substances in your area? How does this compare with the national average?
- Have the Models of Care recommendations been implemented? If not ask your local DAAT commissioner why?
- Who leads on co-ordinating care for pregnant women in your area?

References

Abel EL (1990) *Fetal Alcohol Syndrome.* Oradell, NJ, Medical Economics Company, Inc.

Abel EL, Sokol RJ (1991) A revised conservative estimate of the incidence of FAS and its economic impact. *Alcoholism, Clinical and Experimental Research* 15(3): 514–524.

British Liver Trust website: www.britishlivertrust.org.uk (accessed 5/12/06).

Confidential Enquiry into Maternal and Child Health (CEMACH) (2004) *Why Mothers Die 1997–1999.* London, RCOG.

Day E, George S (2005) Management of drug misuse in pregnancy. *Advances in Psychiatric Treatment* 11: 253–61.

Department of Health (1993) *Changing Childbirth*: report of the Expert Maternity Group (Cumberlege Report). London, HMSO.

Department of Health (2000) *The NHS Plan: a plan for investment, a plan for reform.* London, The Stationery Office.

Department of Health (2004a) *National Service Framework for Children, Young People and Maternity Services.* London, The Stationery Office.

Department of Health (2004b) *Standards for Better Health.* London, The Stationery Office.

Department of Health (2005) *Drug Use, Smoking and Drinking Among Young People in England.* London, The Stationery Office.

Department of Health (2006) *Independent Review of Drug Users.* London, The Stationery Office.

Drug Misuse in Pregnancy Breastfeeding Project (2003) *Breastfeeding and Drug Misuse: An Information Guide For Mothers.* Plymouth, University of Plymouth.

Drugs UK website: www.drugs.gov.uk (accessed 5/12/06).

Drummond DC, Fitzpatrick G (2000) Children of substance misusing parents. In Reder P, McClure M, Jolley A (eds) *Family Matters: Interfaces Between Child and Adult Mental Health.* London, Routledge.

Gossop M, Marsden J, Stewart D, Kidd T (2003) The National Treatment Outcome Research Study (NTORS): 4–5 year follow-up results. *Addiction* 98, 291–303.

Harsch HH, Pankiewicz J, Bloom AS *et al.* (2000) Hepatitis C virus infection in cocaine users – a silent epidemic. *Community Mental Health Journal* 36(3): 225–33.

Healthcare Commission website: www.healthcarecommission.org.uk (accessed 5/12/06).

Hepburn M (1999) Drug use in pregnancy: a multidisciplinary responsibility. *Hospital Medicine* 59(6): 436.

Hepburn M (2005) Social problems in pregnancy. *Anaesthesia and Intensive Care Medicine.* 6(4): 125–26.

Home Office (2003) *Hidden Harm: Responding to the Needs of Children of Problem Drug Users.* London, The Home Office.

Hubbard RL, Craddock, SG, Flynn P *et al.* (1997) Overview of one year outcomes in the Drug Abuse Treatment Outcome Study (DATOS). *Psychology of Addictive Behaviours* 11: 279–93.

Interdepartmental Committee (1961) *Drug Addiction*. The Brain Report, UK.

Interdepartmental Committee (1965) *Drug Addiction, Second Report*. The Second Brain Report, UK.

Kennell JH, Klaus MH (1998) Bonding: Recent observations that alter perinatal care. *Pediatrics in Review* 19(1): 4–12.

Klee H (1997) Illicit Drug Use, Pregnancy and Early Motherhood: An Analysis of Impediments to Effective Service Delivery. Manchester, Manchester Metropolitan University.

MIDIRS (2005) *Alcohol and Pregnancy*. Informed Choice Leaflet No 4. www.infochoice.org/ (accessed 5/12/06).

Mounteney J (1999) *Drugs, Pregnancy and Childcare: A Guide for Professionals*. London, Institute for the Study of Drug Dependence.

National Treatment Agency (2002) *Models of Care for the Treatment of Adult Drug Misusers*. London, NTA.

National Treatment Agency (2006a) *Monthly Drug Statistics in England*. www.nta.nhs.uk (accessed 5/12/06).

National Treatment Agency (2006b) *Models of Care for the Treatment of Adult Drug Misusers*. Update 2006. London, NTA.

Ohto H, Terazawa S, Sasaki N *et al.* (1994) Transmission of Hepatitis C virus from mothers to infants. *New England Journal of Medicine* 330(1): 744–50.

Royal College of Physicians (2001) *Alcohol: Can the NHS afford it?* London, RCP.

Rolleston (1926) Departmental Committee on Morphine and Heroin Addiction, Government Report.

Scottish Executive (2001) A Framework for Maternity Services in Scotland. Scottish Executive.

Scottish Executive (2006) *Integrated Care Pathway For Drug Users*. Scottish Executive.

Shaw NJ, McIvor L (1995) Neonatal abstinence syndrome after maternal methadone treatment. *Obstetrical and Gynecological Survey* 50(7): 511–13.

Simpson D, Sells S (1983) Effectiveness for treatment of drug abuse: an overview of the DARP research programme. *Advances in Alcohol and Substance Abuse* 2: 7–29.

Siney C (2005) *Substance Misuse in Primary Care: A Multidisciplinary Approach*. Oxford, Radcliffe.

Chapter 7
Domestic Abuse in Pregnancy: A Public Health Issue

Sally Price

> Domestic violence is a key issue for the public health agenda. The fact that domestic violence often starts or escalates during pregnancy and is associated with increases in rates of miscarriage, low birth weight, premature birth, fetal injury and fetal death makes for stark reading
>
> (UK Public Health Minister Melanie Johnson 2004)

Introduction

This chapter will help midwives and other health professionals to understand domestic abuse related to pregnancy both in terms of the impact on individuals and the broader public health domain. There is often debate about which is the most appropriate term, abuse or violence. Both terms are powerful and may mean different things to different people, so the terms are deliberately interchanged in this chapter. The effects of abuse on health and pregnancy will be discussed, along with the role of the midwife and the implications for midwifery and public health practice. Current policy and research evidence will be highlighted, combined with an exploration of the psychological and sociological explanations for domestic abuse. It is anticipated that this will result in information that midwives can apply to their own practice and areas of work to promote effective care and services for women and children who live with domestic violence.

Understanding domestic abuse

Many definitions of domestic abuse can be found in the published literature which emphasise the nature of the abuse, and the power and control inequalities that exist in intimate relationships. An accepted example is:

> Domestic violence is any incident of threatening behaviour, violence or abuse, between adults who are or have been intimate partners or family members, regardless of gender or sexuality
>
> (Department of Health 2005)

However, definitions that describe gender inequalities are less common. Despite this, there is no doubt that the vast majority of those who experience domestic abuse are women, with the violence against them inflicted by their former or current male partners. Predisposing factors to domestic violence include marital dependency and lack of economic resources, leading to a higher risk amongst unemployed women or housewives (Walby and Myhill 2000).

Prevalence: key statistics

- At least 1 in 4 women will experience some form of domestic abuse in their lifetime, and 1 in 8 will have repeated experiences.
- Two women are murdered by their current or former partner each week in England and Wales.
- Women between the ages of 16 and 29 are at the highest risk of experiencing domestic violence with an occurrence rate of 28% in women between the ages of 20 and 24.
- Leaving an abusive relationship does not confer protection – 22% of separated women are assaulted by ex-partners (Mirrlees-Black *et al.* 1998).

Caution must be exercised when considering statistical data related to domestic violence. It is well known that domestic violence is vastly under-reported since fear of reprisal and continuing relationships with the perpetrator prevent women from disclosing their experience (Clarkson *et al.* 1994). On average a woman will experience violence up to 35 times before she seeks help (Mirrlees-Black *et al.* 1998). Even when reported the information may not be recorded appropriately, and therefore lost to data collection.

However, British studies are not unique in this failing. From an international perspective, violence against women is often poorly defined, unrecorded or not disclosed, resulting in poor or non-existent services for women. Those studies that do exist show that domestic violence is a worldwide phenomenon, from Japan to Kenya and Germany to Jamaica (Shipway 2004). The World Health Organization has identified how domestic abuse is an infringement of human rights and causes far-reaching damage to the lives and development of individuals and communities (WHO 1997). Across the world domestic violence causes more deaths and disability in women aged 15–44 than cancer, malaria, traffic accidents or war (World Bank Discussion Paper 225 cited by Shipway 2004). Clearly domestic violence is a global public health issue.

Domestic abuse in pregnancy

Domestic abuse has a damaging, and sometimes even life-threatening, impact on the physical and mental well-being of a woman and her baby. Conclusive evidence has demonstrated that pregnancy, far from being a time of peace and safety, may trigger or exacerbate male violence from the home (Royal College of Midwives 1999). Domestic violence is a serious, but often over-looked cause of maternal and infant morbidity and mortality (Drife and Lewis 1998). It is frequently hidden and undisclosed. This makes it difficult to estimate the exact prevalence during pregnancy. However, a recent study by Johnson *et al.* (2003) revealed a prevalence rate of 17%, confirming the findings of several other studies (McFarlane *et al.* 1992; Webster *et al.* 1996). Mezey and Bewley (1997) reported that between 4% and 17% of women disclosed that they were experiencing domestic violence in their current pregnancy. These findings are consistent with the work of McWilliams and McKiernan (1993) who found that 60% of women living in a refuge in Northern Ireland had experienced domestic violence during their pregnancy, with 13% miscarrying their babies as a result of the violence.

Domestic violence is also a significant factor in maternal death as highlighted in the *Why Mothers Die* report 2000–2002. Of the women who died, 14% (n = 51) self-declared before their death that they were subject to violence in the home (CEMACH 2004). In general, women report an increase in the extent and nature of the violence during pregnancy (Dobash 1984). For up to 30% of women who experience domestic violence during their lifetime, the first incident occurs during pregnancy (Helton *et al.* 1987), and 40–60% of women experiencing domestic violence are abused while pregnant (Stark and Flitcraft 1996).

Domestic violence during pregnancy is especially serious, as the health and safety of not one but two individuals are at risk. Pregnant women may experience domestic violence in the same physical ways as those who are not pregnant such as broken bones, bruises, scratches, burns and bites. However there are also some pregnancy-specific effects of domestic abuse, with injuries to the breasts, abdomen and genitalia being more common (Hillard 1985). The risks of miscarriage, placental abruption, antepartum haemorrhage, preterm labour, stillbirth and low birthweight babies are increased (Hillard 1985; Bullock and McFarlane, 1989; Helton *et al.* 1987; Salzman 1990; Mooney 1993). Gynaecological problems such as frequent urinary tract infections, dyspareunia and pelvic pain may also be experienced (RCM 1999). Abdominal trauma to the mother caused by kicking, punching or falling may result in in-utero injuries with fractures to the fetus evident after birth (Mezey and Bewley 1997). Neurological development of the fetus may also be impaired by the adverse effects of hormonal stimulation in response to violent situations experienced by the mother (Shore 1997, cited by Mann 2005).

Physical symptoms related to living with the stress and anxiety of repeated violence may include sleep and appetite disturbances, fatigue, chronic headaches, palpitations, dizziness and even deliberate self-harm as a coping mechanism (RCM 1999). Other coping mechanisms may be adopted with pregnant women who experience domestic violence more likely to use drugs, prescribed and illegal, alcohol and smoking to help them manage living in an abusive relationship (Bhatt 1998). This will have a negative impact on the health of the mother and the growth and development of the fetus. The effect of domestic violence on the mental health of women should not be underestimated. Depression, parasuicide and post-traumatic stress disorder are common in abused women (Golding 1999). Living with domestic violence also shows stronger associations with poor mental health than other experiences of violence, including childhood abuse, sexual abuse and rape (Coid *et al.* 2003). This is of particular significance in pregnancy since psychiatric cases (e.g. suicide) are the leading cause of maternal death (CEMACH 2004).

The impact of domestic violence in pregnancy should not be considered only from the perspective of the mother and fetus. The inter-relationship between domestic violence experienced by the mother and the child must also be considered. Evidence shows that in 33% of child protection cases there is a history of domestic violence and in 55% of known domestic violence cases, children are also being directly abused (Hester and Pearson 1998; Hester *et al.* 1998). The impact of living with domestic violence on babies and children includes maternal infant attachment difficulties, delay in speech and language, difficulties with self-esteem, social competence and peer relationships, greater difficulties with emotional and behavioural development and poorer academic performance (Gonzalez-Doupe 2004). Clearly these difficulties will impact on not only the well-being of the child, but also the mother and any siblings, with long-term consequences for the health of the whole family.

The psychology of abuse

It is important to remember that women who experience domestic abuse are not a homogenous group. They will have varied experiences, feelings, responses and needs. However, the common factor they all experience is the control exerted upon them by the perpetrator including disempowering behaviours such as intimidation, emotional abuse, minimising, denying, blaming, isolation and economic abuse. This may impact on their willingness or ability to seek help. Midwives and other health professionals may fail to recognise this, and may find it difficult to understand why women stay in violent relationships.

The psychology of living in an abusive relationship is complex but Kelly (1999) has identified the six stages that a woman may go through when she lives with abuse.

Explanation	At first she will manage the situation by finding or accepting an explanation for the violence that allows her to continue in the relationship.
Strategies	She may also develop strategies to manage the situation and the abusive incidents.
Make sense	This leads to a distorted perception of the reality of her life, where managing anxiety and trying to make sense of the situation become priorities. At this stage, women view the violence as their responsibility. To cope, she may focus on trying to avoid violence by changing her behaviour.

Realisation	After a number of assaults a woman may come to the realisation that she is a victim of domestic abuse and that some level of responsibility lies with the abuser. Once violence is understood as a recurring feature of her life, she may re-evaluate the relationship and the possibility of leaving becomes easier to consider.
Ending the relationship	Ending the relationship is fraught with difficulties and a woman may return and leave several times. Reasons for this include believing promises of behaviour change, the absence of realistic or practical alternatives, and pressure from others in the family. The lack of effective protection may also be a significant factor, particularly since the risk of death or serious injury is greatly increased around the time of leaving a violent relationship.
Ending the violence	Ending the relationship does not automatically mean the violence will stop. Ending the violence is the sixth and final stage identified by Kelly (1999).

The men who commit domestic abuse have some commonalities. Research has identified that those convicted of domestic violence crimes have disrupted patterns of attachment and high levels of interpersonal dependency and jealousy. They display attitudes that condone violence and often lack empathy. They are also more likely to have witnessed domestic violence as a child. Alcohol was also found to be a major factor in domestic violence offences, with 48% of convicted offenders being alcohol dependent (Home Office 2003). This study also found that perpetrators were likely to fall into one of two groups.

- Borderline emotionally dependent men had high levels of jealousy in stormy intense relationships, with high levels of interpersonal dependence, high levels of anger and low self-esteem.
- Antisocial or narcissistic men tended to have hostile attitudes towards women, low levels of empathy and high rates of alcohol dependency and previous convictions.

Despite this evidence of the altered psychology of men who per-petrate violence and the psychological impact on women of living with abuse, this does not explain why such antisocial behaviour is tolerated and excused. What lies at the root of domestic violence are the gender inequalities promoted and sustained in society.

Domestic violence and society

Living with domestic violence is not a new occurrence for women, although until recently it was considered as a private matter to be held in the domain of the family. In many ways domestic violence towards women is accepted as part of the natural order, with male authority and control and the subordination of women as the social and cultural norm. The family, deemed as a private and sacred institution by the church and the state, maintains and promotes the subordinate position of women. It is this reliance on male partners as a result of a lack of economic independence (as identified by Walby and Myhill 2000) that perpetuates gender inequalities and the subsequent domestic abuse that women and children experience.

Dobash and Dobash (1998) have shown how a conflict of inter-ests in a domestic relationship, based on male status and position in a patriarchal society, can result in violence. Four themes typify this conflict:

- Men's possessiveness and jealousy
- Disagreements related to domestic work and resources
- The acceptability of men's rights to punish women for per-ceived wrongdoings
- The importance of men maintaining power and authority.

Specific issues may act as a source of conflict and trigger the occurrence of violence. These include domestic work, money, children, alcohol, isolation and restriction of social life, and sex. It is not hard to see that in this context pregnancy and the birth of a baby could be a further source of conflict or trigger for violence. The impact of pregnancy on the above issues of conflict may exacer-bate the situation, which may partially explain why, for 30% of women, the first incident of violence occurs during pregnancy (Helton *et al.* 1987).

Gelles (1975) suggests that the normal physiological changes of pregnancy may also act as a trigger for domestic violence. A reduc-tion in libido, combined with hormonal mood swings are given as credible reasons for male violence towards pregnant women. Thus pregnancy can be viewed as interfering with the woman's ability to perform the role ascribed to her by her male partner and this failure to fulfil her 'duty' provokes or justifies a violent response (Price 2003).

These theoretical explanations rely on a perception of women's inability to conform to normal social values as determined by men. As such, this typifies the predominant cultural belief that women are responsible for and deserving of abuse in their intimate relationships. In cases of domestic violence people will often instinctively leap to the defence of the perpetrator (Horley 1991) and try to rationalise or explain the violent behaviour. A further justification for male violence towards women is that women are also often the perpetrators of violence against men. Insisting that domestic abuse is a two-sided issue with women viewed equally as abusers and the abused avoids the reality of the gender inequalities that exist. The overwhelming majority of adults who experience domestic violence are women. The extent of their trauma and injuries is far in excess of that experienced by men (Dobash *et al.* 1995).

The advent of the 21st century has seen a marked change in legislation and policy related to domestic violence. This is largely due to the persistence of organisations such as Women's Aid and Refuge who have worked tirelessly since the 1970s to drive the agenda forward and campaign for radical reform. However, some of the motivation may also have arisen from the huge costs incurred, with domestic abuse draining the resources of public and voluntary services. An evidence-based estimate for the cost of domestic violence has been developed (Walby 2004). In terms of the state, employers and individuals an overall cost of £5.7 billion per year has been found. Within this sum, the cost to the NHS for physical injuries is around £1.2 billion per year, with an additional cost of £176 million for mental health care. By identifying the financial costs, this research gives additional weight to the need for policy interventions to address domestic abuse.

Government policy is driven by an interministerial group that was set up in 2003 and aims to promote a joined up and robust programme of work (Mann 2005) including:

- Increasing safe accommodation choices for women and children
- Improving the interface between criminal and civil law
- Ensuring the police and crown prosecution services respond appropriately
- Promoting education and awareness training
- Developing early and effective health interventions.

The development of early and effective health interventions is vital to the success of supporting the survivors of abuse. Until recently the National Health Service (NHS) has mainly dealt with the physical consequences of domestic violence, with poor pro-active identification. As a result many healthcare organisations have published recommendations promoting the routine enquiry of domestic violence in health and maternity settings (RCM 1999; RCN 2000; DoH 2000; DoH 2005). The Department of Health supports an interagency approach, issuing guidance for healthcare professionals on their role and responsibilities.

The Royal College of Midwives also advocates that every midwife should assume a role in the detection and management of domestic violence (RCM 1999). More recently The Confidential Enquiry into Maternal Deaths in the UK 2000–2002 (CEMACH 2004) has made several key recommendations for maternity services in relation to domestic violence issues in practice. These include the local development of guidelines for the identification of, and provision of support for women who experience domestic violence.

Current changes in legislation include the Domestic Violence Crime and Victims Act 2004, which enforces the protection, support and rights of victims. Work has also been undertaken that has led to the development of a National Plan for Domestic Violence (Home Office 2005) that has five key goals:

- Reducing the prevalence of domestic violence
- Increasing the rate at which domestic violence is reported
- Increasing the rate of domestic violence offences that are brought to justice
- Ensuring the victims of domestic violence are adequately protected and supported nationwide
- Reducing the number of domestic violence-related homicides.

Women's choices and attitudes of carers

Women will rarely voluntarily disclose their abusive experiences, but the use of brief screening questions is known to lead to a higher rate of disclosure, (Bacchus 2002). Research also demonstrates that a majority of women are in favour of routine questioning if asked by a well trained health professional (Bacchus *et al.* 2002). Evidence from the Bristol Pregnancy and Domestic Violence Programme supports this, demonstrating that routine enquiry by well trained and well supported midwives can increase women's disclosure of their experience of abuse (Salmon *et al.* 2004). Routine antenatal enquiry for domestic violence has been endorsed by professional bodies (Royal College of Obstetricians and Gynaecologists (RCOG 2001; RCM 1999), by the Department of Health (DoH 2000; 2005), and recommended by NICE (2003). Ramsey *et al.* (2002) have challenged this view, claiming that implementation of a screening programme in health care settings cannot be justified because of the lack of evidence available of the impact on women or the benefits of specific interventions. This systematic review consists entirely of non-UK based research and did not consider midwifery practice specifically. Nevertheless Ramsey *et al.* (2002) make a valuable contribution to the debate with important questions around routine enquiry into domestic violence in relation to outcomes for women and the role of professionals in undertaking this new extended role.

What is clear is that a key factor in facilitating disclosure from women is the way in which they are asked and the level of support they receive from the person who asks them. This means adopting non-judgmental attitudes, offering women information so they can make informed choices for themselves and their families. Encouraging or cajoling the woman into leaving the abusive relationship may not necessarily have the desired effect of protecting her from the abuser. The riskiest time for experiencing serious violence or death occurs when the woman leaves or attempts to leave the perpetrator (Binney *et al.* 1988; Daly and Wilson 1988). Women who leave will also face huge challenges in terms of finances, accommodation and childcare. However, when women stay in or return to violent relationships they often experience great negativity from health professionals. Comments such as 'well, if it was that bad she'd leave' or 'there's no point, she'll only go back to him,' may be heard. This lack of insight into the reality of women's lives means that professional attitudes and beliefs about domestic violence are biased and unhelpful to those who are surviving it. Other professional attitudes include those who view the women as helpless victims who need saving from their desperate situation. In some respects, this approach simply confirms the power dynamic of the abusive relationship with women seen as passive, weak and disempowered, and unable to act or take responsibility for themselves. At worst, it is yet another form of the patriarchal society controlling women and maintaining their subservient position.

The role of the midwife

Midwives clearly have a role to play in the public health of the nation, and in the context of this chapter that means addressing the domestic violence issues that affect the women they care for. Davis (2005) explains the duality of midwifery practice whereby midwives are able to treat women as individuals, responding to personal circumstances, needs and preferences, yet at the same time manage to consider the impact of environmental, social, political and other lifestyle factors on maternal health. The public health expertise of midwives is further enhanced by their ability to work across the primary and acute sectors of care, ensuring that the pregnancy needs of women are considered in the context of their lives, and not as an isolated medical condition. By practising in this way in both the personal and public spheres midwives can make a valuable contribution to the health and well-being of women who experience domestic violence. This is not to say that this role is easy. On the contrary, it is often difficult, challenging and stimulating, not least because the majority of midwives are women and therefore subject to the same issues related to domestic violence and gender inequalities in their personal and professional lives as the women in their client base.

The role of the midwife in relation to domestic violence can be described under three headings:

- Identification
- Information and support
- Protection and prevention.

Identification

Routine antenatal enquiry to identify domestic abuse is an important aspect of midwifery practice. As previously stated, it is endorsed by professional bodies such as the Royal College of Midwives and is recommended by the Department of Health. On an individual level, asking women about their experiences of violence can make a huge difference to their lives and experience of pregnancy. From a public health perspective, routine enquiry sends a clear message to society as a whole that domestic violence is a health issue and will not be ignored by health professionals.

Asking the question requires an in-depth understanding of this complex subject area. Most midwives are skilled at asking difficult questions of the women they work with, but to ask about domestic violence will require additional training and support, not least because midwives will need to question their own beliefs and attitudes about family violence (Price and Baird 2003). Some may question if indeed it is the midwife's role to ask about domestic abuse. Knowledge of the key risk factors may help, since it has been identified that the main risks are being female, young and poor, which encompasses a large proportion of a midwife's caseload (Baird *et al.* 2004). The impact on health and on pregnancy outlined above also confirms the midwife's role.

Information and support

Midwives need to acknowledge the limitations of their role in relation to domestic abuse. They should not be undertaking a 'search and rescue mission'. Overstepping professional boundaries or becoming personally involved will not be of any benefit. Women should be empowered to take control of their own lives. This may be best achieved by offering information and support to enable women to make informed choices for their future. This may involve leaving the perpetrator, and the midwife will have a role in supporting women to access appropriate services. However, the informed choice that some women will make is to stay in the relationship, and the midwife will need to ensure the woman considers appropriate strategies to promote her safety and that of her children.

It is vital when providing information for women that it is up-to-date and accurate. To give a woman an incorrect or out-of-date telephone number may put her at risk of harm. Working with others is a central component of supporting women who experience violence. Midwives will need to develop interagency and interprofessional relationships to promote this. A sound working knowledge of both local and national resources will help midwives to support women to make the most appropriate choices for their personal circumstances. Midwives should also be mindful of the need to ensure that confidential information does not fall into the hands of the perpetrator, increasing the risk of harm. By seeking advice and working closely with organisations such as the local Women's Aid and the police, midwives and maternity services can ensure that their policies, procedures and practices promote safety and support women's choices rather than increasing risk.

Protection and prevention

Despite the need to promote the empowerment of individuals by supporting their decision making there is a role for midwives to protect and prevent harm to those who live with violence. This may involve working with women to develop a safety plan with means of escape in an emergency, and giving advice about appropriate places of safety and support. It may also include ensuring that documentation not only meets the standards required by the professional body (Nursing and Midwifery Council (NMC) 2002), but also understanding that their records may be used as evidence in court and therefore should also meet the needs of the civil and criminal justice system. Midwifery records or audit may also be used for data collection to inform the public health information base related to the incidence and prevalence of domestic abuse.

There are strong links between domestic violence and child abuse, and a women who is subject to violence herself may be prevented from or unable to protect her children from the damaging effects of witnessing or experiencing violence themselves. The dilemma many midwives face when working with women and children who live with violence is the tension between promoting and supporting informed choices made by the woman and the professional requirement to protect children. Each midwife has the responsibility to safeguard children by acting in a timely and appropriate manner (DoH 2003). This will mean following their organisation's procedures and protocols for promoting and safeguarding children's welfare and knowing who to contact to express and share child protection concerns.

Midwives who are lone workers also need to maintain their own safety. A workplace policy should be available to guide employees on how to reduce personal risks (Unison 2000). This may include:

- Improving systems for information gathering and sharing about patients or clients with a history of violence
- Making arrangements for meeting clients away from their home if a home visit is not essential
- Identification of visits that should not be undertaken in the evening or at night or by a lone worker
- Ensuring that all lone workers leave details of their itinerary and report back to base at regular intervals
- Ensuring that mechanisms are in place to respond if lone worker fails to report back as planned.

Conclusion

Domestic violence is now recognised in the UK as a major public health issue, with serious consequences for maternal and infant health. It affects both the physical and psychological well-being of those who experience it, and has serious implications for long-term individual, family and community health (British Medical Association 1998; James-Hanman 1998). Although domestic violence affects men and women in heterosexual and same-sex relationships, it is a primary cause of gender-specific health inequalities, with female victims far outweighing males. This should be of concern not only to midwives and other health professionals but society as a whole (Baird 2002).

Midwives clearly have a role to play in responding to domestic abuse. Asking women about their experiences of it is accepted as best practice. However, this should not be undertaken in an ad hoc manner with midwives undertaking 'search and rescue' missions, but as part of a considered well structured approach with appropriate support mechanisms for both women and practitioners. In this way midwives and the maternity services can make an effective contribution to tackling domestic violence as both an individual, personal issue and from the perspective of the public health agenda.

Key implications for midwifery practice

- Does your practice include routine enquiry about domestic violence? If not, why?
- Don't be judgmental – appreciate there are many reasons why women stay with their partners.
- Do you know your local domestic violence strategy?
- Can you effectively signpost women who disclose domestic violence to the most appropriate support?
- If you have personal experience of domestic abuse how does this influence your practice?
- Who can provide you with professional support when dealing with cases of domestic violence?

Resources

National Domestic Violence Helpline
0808 2000 247

Women's Aid Federation of England
PO Box 391, Bristol BS99 7SW
0117 944 4411

www.womensaid.org
Provides advice, support and referrals to local refuges, emergency
and temporary accommodation.

Victim Support
Victim Support National Office, Cranmer House, 39 Brixton Road,
London SW9 6DZ
020 7735 9166
www.victimsupport.org.uk
Offers free confidential support and information to people following a crime.

Refuge
2–8 Maltravers Street, London WC2R 3EE
020 7395 700
www.refuge.org.uk
Offers safe temporary accommodation, support and counselling to
women and children suffering from domestic violence.

References

Bacchus L (2002) *Report on the Joint Meeting of the All-Parliamentary Party Group on Maternity and Domestic Violence.* London, RCOG Press.

Bacchus L, Mezey G, Bewley S (2002) Women's perceptions and experiences of routine enquiry for domestic violence in a maternity service. *International Journal of Obstetrics and Gynaecology* 109: 9–16.

Baird K (2002) Domestic violence in pregnancy: a public health concern. *MIDIRS Midwifery Digest* 12(supplement 1): S12–S15.

Baird K, Price S, Salmon D (2004) *The Bristol Pregnancy and Domestic Violence Programme Training Manual.* University of the West of England, North Bristol NHS Trust, Department of Health, Royal College of Midwives. Bristol, University of the West of England.

Bhatt RV (1998) Domestic violence and substance abuse. *International Journal of Obstetrics and Gynaecology* 63(1): 25–31.

Binney V, Harkell G, Nixon J (1988) *Leaving Violent Men: A study of refuges and housing for battered women.* London, Women's Aid Federation of England.

British Medical Association (1998) *Domestic Violence: A Health Care Issue?* London, British Medical Association.

Bullock L, McFarlane J (1989) The battering–low birthweight connection. *American Journal of Nursing* 89(9): 1153–55.

Confidential Enquiry into Maternal and Child Health (CEMACH) (2004) *Why Mothers Die* 2000–2002. London, RCOG Press.

Clarkson C, Cretney A, Davis G, Shepherd J (1994) Assault: the relationship between seriousness, criminalisation and punishment. *Criminal Law Review.* 4 Jan 1994: 4–20.

Coid J, Petruckevitch A, Chung, W *et al.* (2003) Abusive experiences and psychiatric morbidity in women primary care attenders. *British Journal of Psychiatry* 183: 332–39.

Daly M, Wilson M (1988) *Homicide.* New York, Aldine de Gruyter.

Davis K (2005) In O'Luanaigh P, Carlson, C (eds) *Midwifery and Public Health: future directions and new opportunities.* London, Elsevier, pp xi–xii.

Drife J, Lewis G (eds) (1998) *Why Mothers Die: Report on Confidential Enquires into Maternal Deaths in the United Kingdom 1994–1996.* London, HMSO.

Department of Health (2000) *Domestic Violence: A Resource Manual for Health Professionals.* London, DoH.

Department of Health (2003) *The Victoria Climbié Inquiry: report of an inquiry by Lord Laming.* London, The Stationery Office.

Department of Health (2004) *National Service Framework for children, young people and maternity services.* London, The Stationery Office.

Department of Health (2005) *Responding to Domestic Abuse: a handbook for health professionals.* London, DoH.

Dobash RP (1984) The nature and antecedents of violent events. *British Journal of Criminology* 24: 269.

Dobash RE, Dobash RP (1998) *Rethinking Violence Against Women.* London, Sage.

Dobash RE, Dobash RP, Noaks L (eds) (1995) *Gender and Crime.* Cardiff, University of Wales Press.

Gelles R (1975) Violence and pregnancy. A note on the extent of the problem and needed services. *Family Co-ordinator* 24: 81–86.

Golding J (1999) Intimate partner violence as a risk factor for mental health disorders: a meta-analysis. *Journal of Family Violence* 14: 99–132.

Gonzalez-Doupe P (2004) *The Effects of Domestic Violence on Children.* Presentation to the National Domestic Violence and Health Professionals Forum, London, July 2004.

Helton A, McFarlane A, Anderson E (1987) Battered and pregnant: a prevalence study. *American Journal of Public Health* 77(10): 1337–39.

Hester M, Pearson C (1998) *From Periphery to Centre: Domestic Violence in Work with Abused Children.* Bristol, Policy Press.

Hester M, Pearson C, Harwin N (1998) *Making an Impact: children and domestic violence.* Bristol, School for Policy Studies, University of Bristol.

Hillard P (1985) Physical abuse in pregnancy. *Obstetrics and Gynaecology* 66: 185–190.

Home Office (2003) Home Office Findings 217. *Domestic Violence Offenders: characteristics and offending-related needs.* London, The Home Office.

Home Office (2005) *Domestic Violence: a national report.* March 2005. London, The Home Office.

Horley S (1991) *The Charm Syndrome. Why charming men can make dangerous lovers.* London, Paper Mac.

James-Hanman D (1998) Domestic violence: breaking the silence. *Community Practitioner* 71(12): 404–407.

Johnson JK, Haider H, Ellis K, Hay DM, Lindow SW (2003) The prevalence of domestic violence in pregnant women. *BJOG* 110(3): 272–5.

Johnson M (2004) Department of Health press release 20 October 2004 ref 2004/0376 www.dh.gov.uk/PublicationsAndStatistics/PressReleases/PressReleasesNotices/fs/en?CONTENT_ID=4091530&chk=lhOWzZ (accessed 17/12/06).

Kelly L (1999) *Domestic Violence Matters: an evaluation of a development project.* Home Office Research Study 193. London, The Home Office.

Mann C (2005) *Health and Mental Health.* Conference presentation, Domestic Violence and Mental Health in Pregnancy, Imperial College London, November 2005.

McFarlane J, Parker B, Soeken K, Bullock L (1992) Assessing for abuse during pregnancy. *Journal of the American Medical Association* 267: 3176–78.

McWilliams M, McKiernan J (1993) *Bringing it out into the open.* Belfast, HMSO.

Mezey G, Bacchus L, Haworth A, Bewley S (2003) Midwives' perceptions and experiences of routine enquiry for domestic violence. *British Journal of Obstetrics and Gynaecology* 110: 744–52.

Mezey G, Bewley S (1997) Domestic violence and pregnancy. *British Medical Journal* 314(7090): 1295.

Mirrlees-Black C, Budd T, Partridge S *et al.* (1998) *The British Crime Survey: England and Wales.* London, Home Office.

Mooney J (1993) *The Hidden Figures: The North London Domestic Violence Survey.* Middlesex, Middlesex University Centre for Criminology.

National Institute for Clinical Excellence (2003) *Antenatal Care: Routine Care of the Healthy Pregnant Woman.* NICE Clinical Guideline CG006 www.nice.org.uk/guidance/CG6 (accessed 5/12/06).

Nursing and Midwifery Council (2002) *Guidelines for Records and Record Keeping.* London, NMC.

Price S (2003) Domestic violence in pregnancy. In Squire C (ed) *The Social Context of Birth.* London, Radcliffe Medical Press.

Price S, Baird K (2003) Domestic violence: an audit of professional practice. *The Practising Midwife* 6(3): 15–18.

Ramsey J, Richardson J, Carter Y *et al.* (2002) Should healthcare professionals screen for domestic violence? Systematic review. *British Medical Journal* 325(7359): 314.

Royal College of Midwives (1999) *Domestic Abuse in Pregnancy.* Position Paper 19. London, RCM.

Royal College of Nursing (2000) *Position Paper on Domestic Violence.* London, RCN.

Royal College of Obstetricians and Gynaecologists (1997) *Violence Against Women: recommendations arising from study group.* www.rcog.org.uk (accessed 5/12/06).

Royal College of Obstetricians and Gynaecologists (2001) *Why Mothers Die*: Confidential Enquiries into Maternal Deaths in the United Kingdom, 1997–99. London, RCOG.

Salmon D, Baird K, Price S, Murphy, S (2004) *The Bristol Pregnancy and Domestic Violence Programme.* Bristol, University of the West of England, Faculty of Health and Social Care.

Salzman L (1990) Battering during pregnancy: a role for physicians. *Atlanta Medicine* 65: 45–48. In Hunt S, Martin A (eds) (2001) *Pregnant Women, Violent Men: What midwives need to know.* Oxford, Books for Midwives Press.

Shipway L (2004) *Domestic Violence: a handbook for health professionals.* London, Routledge.

Stark E, Flitcraft A, Frazier W (1979) Medicine and patriarchal violence: the social construction of a 'private' event. *International Journal of Health Service* 9: 461–93.

Stark E, Flitcraft A (1996) *Women at Risk: Domestic Violence and Women's Health.* Thousand Oaks, CA, Sage Publications.

Unison (2000) *Working Alone: a health and safety guide on lone working.* London, Unison.

Walby S, Myhill A (2000) *Reducing Domestic Violence: What works? Assessing and managing the risk of domestic violence.* Home Office Briefing Note. London, The Home Office.

Walby S (2004) *The Cost of Domestic Violence.* Key findings. Women and Equality Unit, Department of Trade and Industry. www.womenandequalityunit.gov.uk (accessed 5/12/06).

Webster J, Chandler J, Battistutta D (1996) Pregnancy outcomes and health care use: effects of abuse. *American Journal of Obstetrics and Gynecology* 174: 760–77.

World Health Organization (1997) *Violence Against Women Information Pack: a priority health issue.* Geneva, WHO.

Chapter 8
Maternal Mental Health: Working in Partnership

Samuel Dearman, Kathryn Gutteridge and Waquas Waheed

Depression can be the sand that makes the pearl
(Joni Mitchell, Woman of Heart and Mind 2003)

The minds of mothers

The mental health of women is fundamental to the health of society; it is the pivot upon which the family turns. Women in society have long argued that their health needs are gender-insensitive and this factor is representative in current mental health theories and service provision. Connecting women's mental health to their reproductivity has done little to further this understanding and has raised serious questions about gender differences in health and illness (Astbury 1996). Alongside these issues exists a lack of understanding and acceptance that gender factors are biased in historical research methods, with women's vulnerabilities discounted (Mastroianni *et al.* 1994).

Mental illness in general is highly stigmatised and poorly understood both in society at large and in the healthcare profession. Mental health problems during the childbirth period are relatively common and have far-reaching implications for the health and quality of life for the mother and her family. Mental health issues also significantly complicate other areas of care and represent a large logistical and financial burden for the care of childbearing pregnant women.

This chapter aims to raise awareness of mental illness in the perinatal period, the implications in outcomes for mothers and their children as well as discussing recognition, advice and guidelines for midwives. This focus will draw midwives into the wider public health agenda that is complicated by women's mental health needs.

Epidemiology of perinatal mental illness

Interest in perinatal mental health as a public health issue is escalating. It is a rapidly evolving specialty and specifically concerns women with mental health issues from conception to the end of the first 12 months postpartum (Austin 2004). Psychiatric disorder in pregnancy and following childbirth is common and often serious. Women are not only at risk of relapse of pre-existing mental illness but also at increased risk of suffering new illnesses. The adjustments to childbirth may affect the woman's psychological and social functioning and no matter how positive the birth experience is, it remains a very stressful time for some women.

Global discussions on women's mental health demonstrate a complex picture with poverty, violence and war influential in the development of mental illnesses. There are gender differences and distinctions in women's mental health problems with social positioning, career opportunities, domestic restraints, lifestyle choices and discrimination explaining some of the key issues (Murray and Lopez 1996a). One of the major criticisms of women's health studies is the way that healthcare systems focus on mortality. Saltman (1991) argues that the focus should 'lie in improving morbidity' which in turn will take into context the complexity of women's lives.

The current maternity landscape in the United Kingdom shows that childbirth is safer than ever, with fewer mothers and babies dying. However, childbirth morbidity of women reveals a complex story. The ebb and flow of migrant populations and changes in border agreements with Europe has implications for current service provision and maternal morbidity; these factors will influence care.

Asylum-seeking and refugee status women will bring their own mental health problems, many of them having witnessed war trauma and dealing with grief issues. Those women who have fled their countries to the safety of the United Kingdom may have experienced physical assault and even rape; this has serious implications for their mental well-being and subsequent maternity care. The increased vulnerability of this group of women cannot be underestimated and these factors are inadequately provided for in mainstream maternity and mental health services.

For many women, psychiatric illness occurring during childbirth will adversely affect their quality of life, but also their relationships,

Table 8.1 Incidence of perinatal psychiatric disorder.

Percentage of deliveries	Diagnosis and/or action taken
10%	Postnatal depression
3–5%	Moderate to severe depressive illness
1.7%	Referred to psychiatric services (as a new episode)
0.002%	Admitted with psychosis
0.002%	Admitted with depression
0.002%*	Chronic schizophrenia

Source: Oates (2000).

family and the future development of their children, which will be discussed later in detail. This is not to say that the awareness of mental ill health in the perinatal period is new.

> The incidence of psychiatric illness following childbirth was much greater than the statistics from psychiatric hospitals would indicate and large numbers of cases were cared for at home and never recorded
>
> (Esquirol 1839, cited in Brockington 1996)

There is even reference in the historic texts of Hippocrates, the ancient Greek philosopher who described postpartum psychosis as 'a kind of madness caused by excessive blood flow to the brain and perhaps the overproduction of breastmilk' being a source of mental illness in parturient mothers (Cox 1988).

Women face a clearly established risk of developing a new affective, or mood, disorder during pregnancy and following childbirth (Kendell *et al.* 1987). Table 8.1 shows the approximate percentage of births affected by mental health problems; in the month following childbirth women are at their greatest lifetime risk of referral to psychiatric services (Oates 1994).

Studies from around the world suggest that around 10% of women that have recently given birth will meet diagnostic criteria for a major depressive episode (Spitzer *et al.* 1978). This is elaborated on in the section considering perinatal depression, as the term postnatal depression suggests that the depressive disorder necessarily occurs postpartum, which does not appear to be the case (de Tychey *et al.* 2005). Any type of psychiatric disorder can occur perinatally, and around 20 are described in the literature (Brockington 1996). By far the most common is perinatal depression and the most serious is puerperal psychosis.

Social perceptions and barriers to addressing mental health issues

Mental illness has historically been given negative social connotations. Commonly, mental disorders are not well understood by the general public and indeed healthcare professionals are equally influenced by social perceptions. Stigma in mental health research is an area that has been extensively studied and there is no question that these negative perceptions prevent more satisfactory treatment for people with mental illness.

Stigma occurs in two forms:

Perceived stigma   the negative perceptions of others
Self-stigma   a combination of the individual's own responses and views of mental illness.

Both of these forms of stigma have been considered in research literature.

Perceived stigma

Consistently, studies demonstrate that the media and entertainment industry provide images of people with mental health problems that are distorted and overly dramatic. There has been an overemphasis on criminality, dangerousness and unpredictability, and portrayed social reactions are typified by ridicule, derision, rejection and fear (Stuart 2006). In the literature there are indications that the general knowledge regarding mental health has improved over recent years. However, attitudes towards the mentally ill are inconsistent. A large population-based study has looked at the attitudes of the general public with respect to mental illness, especially the understanding of biological causation. The study concluded that there is still public unease with mental illnesses. However, there is a definite trend towards less perceived stigma, which is particularly pronounced in groups familiar with psychiatric treatment (Angermeyer and Matschinger 2005).

Interestingly, elsewhere different groups have been studied including patients, patients' families, clinicians and the general public examining the attitudes constituting perceived stigma considered key – likelihood of violence, desire for social distance and the causes of illness. Analysis showed that there were no differences between mental health stakeholders and the general public in the likelihood of violence or desire for social distance but there was greater variation between these groups when considering causes of illness. Throughout the analysis the researchers found that it was the clients themselves that tended to have the most negative views of illness (Van Dorn *et al.* 2005).

Childbearing is a complex shift in psychological transition from one psychodynamic state to another; this has great implications for women. There are elements of loss and attachment deficits for childbearing women; this encompasses social repositioning, body image changes, boundary breaches and disappointment (Raphael-Leff 2001). Some of the symptoms of postnatal depression – shame, guilt, secrecy and stigma – reveal how women experience their mental health and this in itself may prevent women from accessing healthcare and treatment.

There is also a great deal of mythology around mental health and motherhood, 'They will take my baby away from me' being a classic example. This demonstrates how a woman may fear engagement with health services and how she may be perceived as a failure in society's eyes.

Self-stigma and self-esteem

The effects of the perceived stigma of mental illness can be thought as causing some of the impaired self-esteem widely reported by people with mental illness (Stuart 2006). This self-stigma adversely influences the individual at the level of their illness and affects their engagement with mental health services.

In the literature, health-seeking behaviour has been examined in different groups of people with mental health problems. Quite understandably, as a consequence of the perceived stigma patients are embarrassed about seeking professional help and expect to encounter a negative reaction even if they do so, both from the health professionals and the general public. The combination of this expectation of negative reactions and embarrassment reduce the likelihood of health-seeking from mental health professionals (Das *et al.* 2006; Barney *et al.* 2006). These effects also reduce an individual's adherence to medication and hence overall recovery and reduce well-being, creating morbidities and mortalities that are preventable and treatable (Gary 2005). Role modelling by media, inclusive public involvement and continued midwifery input and support are excellent ways to normalise mental illness and motherhood.

Future of stigma in mental healthcare management

Even given some of the inconsistency in the research literature, few would contest that directly addressing problems in the area of stigma is necessary in the approach to mental healthcare.

Recently, innovative research has considered what role screening and intervention may have in identifying those individuals who are particularly vulnerable to the effects of stigma. Work from the US has indicated that the use of assessment scales could be used to determine those most in need of education and support to increase their likelihood of accessing mental health services (Bambauer and Prigerson 2006). As mentioned above, the portrayal of mental health problems tends towards negative beliefs and reactions in the media and entertainment industry. Although in its early stages, the effects of Entertainment–Education strategies (Ritterford and Jin 2006), specifically about schizophrenia, have been studied to examine the role of knowledge acquisition in stigma reduction. Viewing an accurate and empathic movie portrayal can increase knowledge of mental illness and the use of an educational trailer increased knowledge and influenced stigma reduction. At this stage, measures specifically targeting causes and problems of mental health stigma do not form a part of management but remain an area of interest in research.

Understanding maternal mental illness, its causes and the way it is experienced is both necessary and vital to ensure that women, their families and society are aware of the consequences these illnesses wreak both in the short and longer term. It is important to begin with pregnancy and examine how this emotional journey can be the precipitating factor for some women to experience mood lability and the subsequent descent into a range of mental illnesses.

Antenatal depression

The confirmation of pregnancy is not necessarily supported by joyful feelings and great anticipation. The 'blue line' of a positive pregnancy test may be a trigger for anxiety and mood changes that many women fail to disclose to even their closest family. This burden of negativity can lead to internalisation and guilt feelings with depression being one of the consequences.

Antenatal depression itself is a little understood phenomenon. In one study, 23% of all women with postnatal depression disclosed that their symptoms had started during pregnancy (Murray *et al.* 1996). Further studies revealed that depression in pregnancy has strong association with:

- Poor attendance at antenatal clinic
- Substance misuse
- Low birthweight
- Premature births (Cox *et al.* 1982; Watson *et al.* 1984; Wilson *et al.* 1996; Evans *et al.* 2001).

It was a commonly held view that depression was minimal during pregnancy and a protective factor. However, recent evidence shows risks are potentially higher (Murray and Lopez 1996b; Evans *et al.* 2001). Evidence shows there is no correlation with antenatal depression and the manifestation of postnatal depression, with most women who are depressed during pregnancy finding their symptoms lift during the postpartum period (Cox *et al.* 1993).

Many other mental health problems are often hidden from daily life but may exacerbate during the childbirth year – eating disorders, self injurious behaviours, compulsive behaviours, unhealthy coping methods such as substance misuse and a range of anxiety-based disorders are just a few (WHO 2000).

The impact of maternity care during pregnancy offers reassurance for some women but it may be anxiety-provoking for others. The establishment of a trusting relationship with a midwife can help to ameliorate some of the normal anxieties and should not be underestimated in its importance. Often women value the confiding nature of this relationship and where other health professionals fail to engage, midwives are more successful in accessing both information and health changes.

Case study: valuing the mother–midwife relationship

Cara is pregnant with her second baby and is meeting with her midwife for the first time. She is anxious and unhappy about the pregnancy. During the booking history session, Cara starts to cry and discloses to her midwife she is feeling 'quite low' and does not know if she really wants this baby. Her first son is two years old, and she feels as if she is just starting to get her life back together. The birth of her first child was not an experience she enjoyed, she hated her changing body and she also felt 'strange' when her baby started to move. She felt particularly frightened about the onset of labour and the birth was long with interventions. Cara has also just got a job she really wanted and is enjoying the extra responsibility placed upon her.

> The midwife listens attentively and encourages Cara to share her anxieties. Cara feels as if she has shared her burden and values the time the midwife has given her. The midwife makes a note in her hand-held records about her anxiety and discusses this with the GP and health visitor; they monitor Cara's progress through the pregnancy. The team give Cara information about yoga antenatal classes and the aromatherapy service at her birth centre.

Baby blues

It is important to distinguish depressive disorder from 'baby blues', which is a relatively normal occurrence tending to be short-lived and self-limiting between 3–5 days postpartum. The association with the onset of lactation and the combination of postnatal weariness mean that women experience varying levels of tearfulness and anxiety.

Although distressing, 'baby blues' is not an interchangeable term with depression and this emotional lability is reported in between 26–85% of women depending on how it is measured (Whiffen 1991). It is important that women understand the nature and duration of this transitional emotional stage; their anxieties and feelings should be validated rather than dismissed. Early transfer home has not been associated with exacerbation of 'baby blues'. but if mothers are separated from their infants, who may be cared for in neonatal services, separation anxiety may be a feature (Forman *et al.* 2000).

The onset of 'baby blues' often coincides with lactational engorgement; this can be a difficult time for women to manage and endure. It is important that women receive support, encouragement and expert advice from midwives and other healthcare workers in establishing breastfeeding that does not complicate the lability of their mood.

Whereas 'baby blues' is shortlived and to a greater degree expected, this differs from postnatal depression, which is a syndrome of low mood lasting for at least two weeks with a constellation of biological, cognitive and emotional symptoms.

Postnatal depression

Depression following childbirth is insidious, often unexpected by women and potentially serious for a number of mothers. A recent systematic review and meta-analysis of the literature has considered the incidence and prevalence of perinatal depression in order to produce reliable rates (Gavin *et al.* 2004). In terms of prevalence, the number of cases at any one time, the authors concluded that up to 18.4% of women will suffer depression, with as many as 12.7% having an episode of major depression. As many as 19.2% of mothers may go on to have major or minor depression in the first three months postpartum.

In terms of incidence, the number of new cases, 14.5% of pregnant women will have a new episode of depression and 14.5% following childbirth. Figures for major depression were 7.5% and 6.5% respectively (Gavin *et al.* 2004).

Any mental health problem will have significant impact upon a woman's ability to cope with the extra demands of pregnancy and mothering. Early identification, the availability of appropriate and timely interventions and support, with effective interagency approaches to service delivery, are essential elements of good mental health support during pregnancy and childbirth (DoH 2002). There is little evidence to support the prevention of postnatal depression, but the current research base for preventive interventions in low-risk women is limited and inconclusive (Tully *et al.* 2002).

The manifestations of symptoms are generally seen within 4–6 weeks postnatally, but some women will present much later into the postnatal period. Low mood, changes in sleep and appetite, loss of interest, anxiety states, feeling guilty and ashamed are just some of the ways a woman will present. There are those women, however, whose depression will be at the severe end of the spectrum and who need admission to a mother and baby unit. It is important that specialist services work with midwives to ensure that normality is maintained and that the relationships a woman forges with her midwife continue (Nursing and Midwifery Council (NMC) 2004).

Puerperal psychosis

Puerperal psychosis is a serious disorder consisting of psychotic symptoms, mood symptoms (depression or mania) and commonly disorientation. Puerperal psychosis occurs in the first six weeks following childbirth, often starting within the first week. Around 2 per 1000 women delivered are admitted to hospital with puerperal psychosis (Oates 2000) and it is at this time in women's lives that they are at their most vulnerable to psychosis, as demonstrated in Figure 8.1.

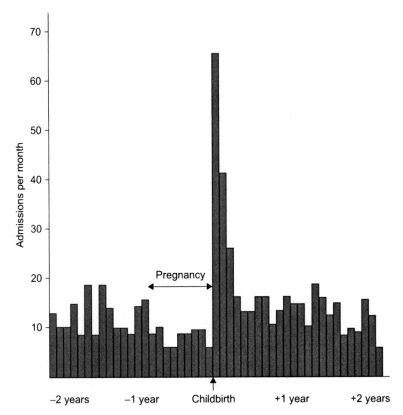

Figure 8.1 Rate of admission of women with psychosis.
Adapted from Kendell et al. (1987).

If puerperal psychosis is suspected, sensitive questions about the woman's ideas or plans of harming herself or her baby should be pursued without exception. It is also important to consider safeguarding of the child in the presence of puerperal psychosis. Referral to social services may be required to support the mother and her baby.

A woman can expect to be transferred home from a hospital birth within hours of her baby being born. This has implications for the midwifery care she will receive at home. Many of the symptoms of puerperal psychosis may display a similar picture to the emotional lability of the 'baby blues' so distinction and definition are imperative for both the mother and her baby.

Midwives who encounter a woman with puerperal psychosis may need advice and support themselves, as being with a woman who is psychotic is disturbing to witness. The family often turns to health professionals for advice and support, which can be

demanding. Talking with colleagues, discussing with expert practitioners and with supervisors of midwives is a healthy way to
reflect upon how it feels to support the woman and her family.

Post-traumatic stress disorder (PTSD) and traumatic birth

Whereas postnatal depression and puerperal psychosis have
received increased public interest and acceptability, there still
remains a reluctance to address and understand the issues associated with post-traumatic stress and childbirth. This phenomenon
is commonly dismissed and little understood in the main.

The International Classification of Disease 10 (ICD-10) recognises
PTSD as a significant mental health determinant and, using
criteria from the *Diagnostic and Statistical Manual of Mental Disorders Fourth Edition* (DSM-IV), is the standard by which diagnosis
is made (American Psychiatric Association 1994; World Health
Organization 1992).

Although in the first instance PTSD was largely synonymous
with war and hostage situations there has been a broadening of the
definition, which now includes childbirth. NICE (2005) produced
guidance for PTSD and considers childbirth to be a significant
stressor which places some women at risk of developing the full
range of PTSD symptoms. Ryding *et al.* (1998) report that it is possible to identify factors that may predispose a woman to develop
PTSD; these include unexpected caesarean section; prolonged
exposure to labour with inadequate pain relief; and hostile staff.

The prevalence of PTSD following childbirth is reported to be
between 2–7% and data collected by the Birth Trauma Association
(BTA) (2006) state that as many as 10 000 women in the UK have
the full constellation of symptoms to be diagnosed. The emotional
experience of birth and the primal nature of labour are potential
stressors (Olde *et al.* 2006). Empirical evidence confirms that childbirth can lead to the development of a PTSD profile. Olde *et al.* (2006)
further report that among identified risk factors were a history of

> . . . psychological problems, trait anxiety, obstetric procedures,
> negative aspects in staff–mother contact, feelings of loss of con-
> trol over the situation, and lack of partner support
>
> Olde *et al.* (2006)

Many women do not have their symptoms recognised and
many receive a general diagnosis of postnatal depression, which
delays treatment and recovery (Beech and Robinson 1985). The

experience of trauma during childbirth has implications for maternal–infant attachment and will influence the relationship a woman has with her newborn baby. If the symptoms are unrecognised and left untreated, it is probable that the woman will go on to develop enduring health problems (Beck 2004). Beck (2004) describes PTSD and childbirth as a combination of 'objective and subjective factors'; these include mode of delivery and feelings of loss of control and dignity. When describing their childbirth experiences women with PTSD will use language that is often heard in the same context as torture or rape victims.

Many maternity units have developed birth reflection and birth debriefing services for postnatal women with anxiety and trauma symptoms. Small *et al.* (2006) invite caution; in their research looking at outcomes of a midwife-led trial of debriefing for women who experienced an operative birth, they found at six months postpartum that there was no benefit of debriefing in improving maternal mental health outcomes. However, one of the findings of concern is the possibility that debriefing may have contributed to emotional health problems in the intervention group. This prompted longer-term follow-up of participants (Small *et al.* 2000).

It is considered vital that debriefing does not traumatise, minimise or exist for the purpose of deflecting complaints; if it is to be done, it should be carefully managed by appropriately trained individuals. Supervision of counselling and debriefing is important and differs from traditional midwifery supervision. Input from psychology and psychotherapy is immensely useful.

Policy drivers

In 2000 the government launched the NHS Plan putting patients at the heart of healthcare service delivery (DoH 2000). This plan identified those areas of health that suffered from lack of resources and poor access to services; mental health was acknowledged as such. This policy also stated that public representation and consultation should be at the centre of decision making about local healthcare. This plan led the way for many other policies and principles of care to be developed with the emphasis upon equality and accessibility of high quality care.

Women's Mental Health: Into The Mainstream (DoH 2002) outlined in detail the separate areas of women's mental health, identifying the recognised epidemiology, interventions and areas of good practice. In the document there is evidence of the acknowledgement of the scale of problems faced regarding perinatal mental health and proactive approaches to solutions. To a limited extent the midwife is acknowledged as having a role in perinatal mental health but the document has been criticised for not being sufficiently holistic, and not referring to the wider implications for families (Currid 2004).

In 2003 the Department of Health published its analysis of responses to the consultation questions posed in *Women's Mental Health: Into the Mainstream* (DoH 2003). There was a general feeling that there is a need for a larger evidence base and that information should be effectively disseminated through clinical governance, new letters and local education. Opinion suggested that patients could be involved in commissioning services. With specific reference to perinatal mental health there was again a call for an increased evidence base, that postnatal depression should be used as a specific term, specialist units and further training are needed and that a more implicit emphasis should be put on the impact of perinatal mental health problems on their children.

While it is important that policies force the issues, it is imperative that women and their families are included in any of the local and national decision-making processes. Bringing maternity services together in a way that engages health workers and public representation is the work of maternity services liaison committees. In all areas, these committees will consider and influence the local needs of childbearing women and their infants; some produce information for new parents and what they may expect during the childbirth period.

Another document influential in women's mental health needs is the *National Service Framework for Children Young People and Maternity Services* (DoH 2004). This important publication builds upon *Every Child Matters* and the principles of children's well-being being integral to their parent's health (DfES 2004).

Guidelines produced by the National Institute of Clinical Excellence (NICE) are generally accepted as the gold standard for guidance in the UK. Long-awaited guidelines for antenatal and postnatal mental health issues were published by NICE in January 2007 as this book was going to press, and reference is made to maternal mental health problems in the recent publication of the postnatal care guideline (DeMott *et al.* 2006).

The triennial report *Why Mothers Die* has done much to raise attention on the nature and outcomes of women who have died with a psychiatric illness (CEMACH 2004). The elaboration of mental illness and the deconstruction of events leading to the deaths of women, many who committed suicide have raised concerns about the lack of insight in this area (Robinson and Beech

1991). In the latest report there were a significant number of women who had contact with a range of healthcare professionals and yet the depth of their distress was not discovered until after their deaths (CEMACH 2004).

Suicide kills more mothers than hypertensive disease, yet it receives far less attention as a cause of maternal death (Robinson 1998). Between 2000 and 2002 severe mental illness caused or contributed to 60 maternal deaths due to suicide in the UK (RCOG 2001). Mental illnesses were reported to be the second most common cause of death in the Late Indirect category. However, the report identifies difficulties in reporting exact numbers due to under-reporting. Suicide during the childbirth period has some interesting distinctions to non-childbearing women. It is significant that pregnancy has some protective factors that prevent suicidal intent, but risk of suicide is still significant for some women. A profile derived from the Confidential Enquiries into Maternal Deaths (CEMACH 2004) showed that women who die in violent circumstances are more likely to:

• be white
• have more than one child
• be over the age of 25
• be married and living in comfortable circumstances
• be educated
• have previous mental health diagnosis
• be in late pregnancy trimester or within 12 weeks postpartum.

Crosscultural studies find little difference with prevalence and symptom manifestation of perinatal illness. In 1990, women of childbearing age completing suicide in China amounted to 180 000; diagnosis of mental illness was an underlying factor in those deaths (WHO 2000). It is imperative that midwives understand the prevalence and profile of these women's choice of death to risk assess and implement preventive strategies.

Midwives, mothers and screening for mental illness

Midwives are ideally placed to provide early detection of perinatal mental illness. As mentioned previously, the last two triennial reports (RCOG 2001; CEMACH 2004) highlighted the need to improve the care of women with mental health problems in the perinatal period, with midwives contributing largely to the detection and recognition of such women.

Table 8.2 Recommendations for midwifery practice in perinatal psychiatric disorder.

- At the first 'booking' visit specific enquiries should be made regarding previous episodes of mental illness in a sensitive and systematic manner.
- In the case of women with a history of long and enduring/severe mental health problems a referral to a psychiatrist should be made with a view to establishing an agreed management plan, due to the risks of recurrence.
- The term postnatal depression or PND should be considered a specific term and not be used generically in the description of other types of mental illness.

Source: CEMACH (2004).

The Confidential Enquiry; Why Mothers Die (CEMACH 2004) made some key recommendations in relation to midwifery practice, summarised in Table 8.2.

Perinatal mental health care may be overly reliant on the Edinburgh Postnatal Depression Scale (EPDS) (Cox *et al.* 1987) and standard approaches have been criticised elsewhere (Shakespeare 2001), as a significant number of women with perinatal psychiatric disorder continue to go undiagnosed by primary healthcare professionals (Hearn *et al.* 1998).

Central to the recommendations of this report (RCOG 2001) is the need for adequate assessment and documentation at the initial booking visit by midwives aiming for information about mental health issues. The booking visit establishes the relationship between midwife and mother whereby risks can be assessed; the likelihood of recurrence of previous perinatal mental illness or of familial factors allows the midwife to identify those women at greater risk.

Midwives can subsequently support women through the process of referral to psychiatric services and jointly work together agreeing a plan of management. Those women with a history of perinatal mental health problems together with those with a history of non-perinatal mental health problems should be considered particularly at risk (Wieck *et al.* 1991).

Other risk factors relating to social adversity and lifestyle, e.g. substance misuse, should also be considered when making an assessment of risk (DoH 1999; Hart *et al.* 2001). The prompt and appropriate referral of at-risk women to psychiatric services would improve the quality of care for most women, indeed it has been claimed that deaths may be prevented (Oates 2001).

Example of good practice: assessing risk

Angela is pregnant with her first child attending the booking visit. The midwife asks Angela about her past medical history. Angela tells the midwife she has been diagnosed with bipolar disorder and was taking regular medication until her pregnancy was confirmed. When asked about her family Angela revealed her grandmother had 'gone mad' after each of her two pregnancies and had electroconvulsive therapy. Angela told the midwife she was very scared of the same thing happening to her and that she might have her baby 'taken away'.

Angela's midwife reassured her and made a referral to the perinatal liaison service and told her she and other skilled health workers would continue to see her throughout the pregnancy. Angela was given information about local services provided to mothers and their babies for support after birth. The midwife communicated this information to Angela's GP, health visitor, obstetrician and midwifery colleagues in both hospital and community.

Whether midwives are fully prepared to take on the responsibility of eliciting an adequate psychiatric history and properly preparing women for the possibility of future mental illness has been questioned. Central to the argument in the content of the midwife's assessment is what actually constitutes an adequate psychiatric risk assessment, but this has not formally been agreed and surveys suggest that further training is needed (Stewart and Henshaw 2002). This sets the precedent for specific training for student midwives in the preregistration period.

The subject as to whether or not community psychiatric nurses (CPNs) are best placed to manage women with perinatal psychiatric disorder has been debated (Hanley 1998). In general, services are set up in such a way that the role of the CPN is more directed towards the management of people with enduring mental illness, and it could be suggested that without further training there is little evidence to promote CPNs taking a primary role in supporting expectant mothers with perinatal mental health problems.

Supporting women in promoting mental health

Good midwifery practice is key in the facilitation of childbearing women and new mothers to feel supported and positive during pregnancy and postpartum (Church and Scanlan 2002). Midwives may even help to prevent depression in the perinatal period (Kumar *et al.* 1995). Midwifery may be thought of as providing a continuum of support from pregnancy to the postnatal period; this is achieved with education, support and prompt effective referral.

Midwives are often described as advocates for women, with skills in asking difficult questions and making hard decisions about referring women to social services when the unborn child may be at risk. The relationship that forms between a woman and her midwife can be a key factor in observing mood changes during pregnancy – after the birth it should not be underestimated in providing timely and effective interventions.

New evidence continues to demonstrate the need for effective, appropriate assessment underpinned by good communication, but the reality is often lacking. It remains clear that the midwife is in a unique position as the first point of contact throughout pregnancy as part of interdisciplinary integration (Halbreich 2005), and it is reassuring that effective screening programmes are achievable in the context of busy clinics (Thoppil *et al.* 2005). It remains an issue of debate whether midwives should have a role in the perinatal mental health team or continue with conventional midwife teams working in partnership with other professions.

Midwives are able to support women in promoting continuity of care during perinatal mental health management (Bindman *et al.* 2000). Midwife support can extend beyond the traditional 28 days, preventing the need for women to have to repeat their history and current problems; allowing the process to be less traumatic; reducing the contact with perceived stigma and likelihood of disengagement (Church and Scanlan 2002). This midwifery approach aims to assist women in feeling 'normal' (Douglas and Arias 2002). Pregnant women may fear stigmatisation following referral to a mental health worker, such as a community psychiatric nurse, but there is less stigma associated with contact with professionals within maternity care (Parkes and Hardy 1997). Ross-Davie *et al.* (2006) found that although midwives are willing to develop their public health role in relation to mental health, they often lack training and confidence in the area.

The midwife has a vital role in assessing and supporting women with perinatal mental health problems and the development of future perinatal mental health services. There must be an emphasis on collaborative working and communication with sensitive and specific focus on mental health problems at the first point of contact.

Management of serious perinatal illness

In 1992 the Royal College of Psychiatrists established a group focusing on postnatal mental illness. It published a council report recommending that a consultant psychiatrist should treat women requiring secondary psychiatric services with a special interest in the condition with the support of a multidisciplinary team (MDT). Inpatient care was advocated, if required, together with the baby, and where available in a specialist unit. In 1996 the Royal College of Psychiatrists formed a joint advisory group with the Department of Health.

Based on the 1992 report, advice for service provision specifically for childbearing women was produced. However, this was delayed in 1996 due to the change of government and healthcare policy at that time. Since then, the advisory group has published the 2000 Council Report CR88 (RCPsych 2000) suggesting that because perinatal psychiatric disorder is common, potentially serious and has long-standing effects on both mother and child, every health authority should have a perinatal mental health strategy. This strategy should aim to make knowledge, skills and resources available such that prompt detection and effective treatment are in place at all levels of healthcare provision.

The advice suggests that a consultant psychiatrist with a special interest in perinatal psychiatric disorder be identified who would take the lead in promoting aims and in establishing a specialist MDT. All women with perinatal psychiatric disorder requiring psychiatric care should have access to this MDT, irrespective of their place of residence. The advisory group was of the view that mother and baby units should be established that would serve the needs of a number of health authorities. The need for communication has been strongly emphasised and the MDT framework considered key. Effective liaison should occur not only with primary care and other psychiatric services but also with midwives, health visitors and obstetricians. Skills and communication would need to be available across many settings – not only inpatient units but also outpatient departments and the community.

When producing policies for the provision of service a cost benefit analysis is inevitable. The advisory group used the critical mass argument to justify the need for specialisation using data regarding the population at risk. It is true that midwives and health visitors care for young mothers and their families almost exclusively; with training they can manage many common mental health problems with the assistance of GPs (Appleby *et al.* 1997).

In a psychiatric sector that services a population of 100 000 with an annual birth rate of 1200 (approximately) there would be expected to be around 25 referrals per year. Of these, only two may have psychosis. Logistically, it would be problematic for staff to maintain skills and hence provide effective safe service. However, if the health authority area as a whole were considered, a sufficient number of referrals would be expected that would then justify specialist community teams and consultant psychiatrist sessions.

Existing service provision

In the UK there are few specialist units or community teams. For some time now, health visitors and midwives have been trained in the use of the EPDS and in many areas they have been trained in non-directive counselling and cognitive-behavioural approaches.

Numerous national initiatives also include projects in perinatal mental health, Sure Start being an example. There are assessment and treatment residential units in the UK that are both voluntary and statutory social services. These are staffed by specialist social workers and do not cater specifically for mothers with mental illness. Funding comes from social services.

Voluntary organisations such as Home-Start, Association for Postnatal Illness (APNI) and the National Childbirth Trust (NCT) have long supported women and their families in the community. Many women have found support and comfort in meeting with other women with postnatal depression and have come through their illness often without mainstream intervention.

Example of good practice: a social model of support

'Mums in Mind' is a model of support working with Home-Start and offering a therapeutic framework enabling women to examine their feelings in relation to their postnatal depression. The facilitation is semi-structured and co-facilitated with a midwife, health visitor, Home-Start co-ordinator and visiting counsellor. The aims are to raise general awareness, share stories and experiences but also to educate women around the impact of living with a range of perinatal mental health problems. The group meets weekly and the women are referred to the group by health visitors, midwives, GPs, family and even friends. The mothers are invited along and given a written card of what they might expect, they are asked to place their children in the crèche provided so they are less likely to be distracted from the discussions. The group is based upon the Tamworth Postnatal Depression Support Group, which was first launched in 1997 and is still successfully running (Gutteridge 2002).

Media public figures such as Fern Britton have done a great deal to raise awareness of postnatal mental illness; this often has more significant impact than professional bodies in persuading government policy change. In addition, Internet access can give women reassurance and contact with other women during their illness, for example, the Association of Postnatal Illness (APNI).

While there is no doubt that women with serious mental health problems require specialist care, voluntary organisational help is vital to other women with mild to moderate depression. However, there remain large areas across the UK where no such services exist.

Service framework for perinatal services

The relief of suffering and promotion of maternal and infant well-being are considered a valid reason for intervention. It is acknowledged that midwives, child welfare services, primary care, social services and the voluntary sector, can manage less serious conditions.

The specifics of a service are influenced by a number of factors. The Royal College of Psychiatrists suggests that evidence from original research and best clinical practice should form the core standards of care that determine what services are delivered to patients. However, service frameworks must also take into account local considerations such as birth rate, economics, sociodemography and the existing framework of mental health service delivery (Figure 8.2).

A framework of three tiers is suggested that would work as a hierarchy to this. It would aid integration and communication and prevent services being duplicated (Figure 8.3).

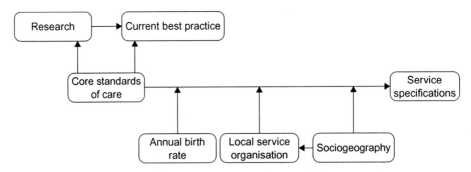

Figure 8.2 The influence of core standards and local considerations in perinatal mental health service delivery.
Source: Oates (2000).

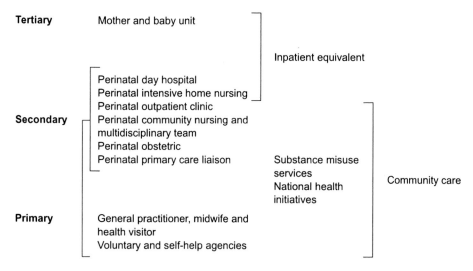

Figure 8.3 A service framework for perinatal mental health.
Source: Oates (2000).

The Royal College of Psychiatrists advisory group summarises its core standards as follows:

- Health authorities should have a strategy for the care of women with perinatal psychiatric disorders at all levels of healthcare provision.
- Women who experience perinatal psychiatric disorders should have access to suitable treatments at the appropriate level of healthcare.
- Women with perinatal psychiatric disorders should have access to a consultant psychiatrist with a special interest supported by professionals with experience and skills in this area.
- Women requiring admission for perinatal psychiatric disorders should be admitted to specialist mother and baby units.

The effects of perinatal mental illness on future generations

Studies considering the impact of perinatal mental health problems on the children have quite consistently reported a variety of adverse effects. A body of evidence has been collected over the years that demonstrates perinatal ill health in the mother has implications for the child's emotional, cognitive and physical development, although there is much less literature regarding the latter. The focus in research has been on the effects of depression and it is this that shall be discussed here. In this section we will consider development in infancy and early childhood with specific reference to emotional and cognitive development and later consider the physical aspects.

Development in infancy

While observing depressed mothers' face-to-face interactions with their infants a number of studies of 3–6-month-olds have found that the children show fewer positive facial expressions, more negative expressions, more protest behaviour, more drowsiness and fussiness, less relaxation and contentment, decreased physical activity and vocalisations (Field *et al.* 1984, 1985, 1988). An often quoted study showed that infants aged 6–7 months of depressed mothers displayed certain recognised insecure behaviour, that of insecure-avoidance (Cohn *et al.* 1986).

It must be noted that not all evidence has been consistent and that in some studies little or no differences were found between infants of depressed and non-depressed mothers (Campbell *et al.* 1995; Murray 1992; Murray *et al.* 1996). The socioeconomic status in these studies was considered and it has been concluded that when there is no wider social disadvantage, no association is found between depression in the mother and disturbed infant interactions; but where such disadvantage is present, infants will show a range of disturbed behaviours.

When infants have been studied independently from their mothers there remain reports of disturbed behaviour at three months of age, accompanied by increased maternal reports of infant crying, confirmed by direct observations (Cutrona and Troutman 1986). In this area infants are more tense, less content and tend to deteriorate more quickly when exposed to stress (Whiffen and Gotlib 1989).

At 12–18 months of age, clear abnormalities in cognitive development have been demonstrated. Using recognised measures of cognitive development, infants of depressed mothers are less developed in mental and motor skills and tend to fail tasks of object permanence (i.e. the conceptual ability to comprehend of an object's existence when no longer visible) achieved by infants of the same age with mothers who are not thought to be depressed. For example, at three days old an infant will recognise its mother and prefer her to others, but does not become distressed when she leaves the room; this changes as the child's cognitive development matures and at around eight months the infant will experience degrees of anxiety and distress when separated from its mother even for short periods of time.

This appears to hold true irrespective of the mother's intelligence quotient (IQ) and is more of an area of concern in boys (Murray *et al*. 1996).

Emotional development, studied in a number of ways, has also been shown to be different in later infancy in the presence of maternal depression. For infants of depressed mothers there appears to be less affective sharing (or mood sharing), less interaction, poorer concentration and increased negative responses. These seem to persist after the mother's depression is resolved. Previously mentioned, insecure-avoidance attachment styles also persist at age 18 months (Lyons-Ruth *et al*. 1986; Murray 1992) but not all studies confirm this observation (Campbell and Cohn 1996). The depressed mothers have been found to report behaviourally difficult children with more temper tantrums, sleeping or eating problems and attachment anxiety.

It is important that midwives understand the detrimental effect of attachment disorders and the need to establish strong maternal–infant attachment as soon after birth as possible. Establishing breastfeeding is an important factor in this mother–infant relationship and the impact of 'skin to skin' for all babies regardless of feeding choice is a crucial aspect of beginning this bond.

Development in childhood

By 4–5 years of age, children of depressed mothers perform significantly lower on tests of general cognitive development and this again seems to be more the case in boys and may be confined to cases where the mother is less well educated (Cogill *et al*. 1986; Hay and Kumar 1995; Sharp *et al*. 1995). However, as stated earlier, one longitudinal study (Murray *et al*. 1996) failed to demonstrate delayed cognitive development or milestones. More recent research suggests that, in fact, demonstrably lower IQ may be present in children of 11 years of age (Hay *et al*. 2001).

In terms of emotional functioning, a clear pattern has yet to be established in later childhood. Some studies have suggested raised levels of child disturbance but they did not continue to statistical significance (Ghodsian *et al*. 1984; Wrate *et al*. 1985; Caplan 1989). However, boys of depressed mothers are significantly less mature in early childhood than girls of depressed mothers when rated by teachers (Sinclair and Murray 1998).

There is increasing evidence that maternal depression is implicated in a range of cognitive and emotional abnormalities and delays, particularly in boys. Maternal–infant interactions can be an influential denominator in the long-term social and cognitive development of children – this is further complicated when additional phenomena are present in women's lives such as social factors, family health problems and deprivation which co-exist with a depressive episode following the birth of a child.

The physical development of children with depressed mothers

The effects of maternal perinatal ill health on the physical development of children have been under-researched. In utero development may be affected by hormones in the hypothalamic pituitary adrenal axis, the hormones involving growth and stress responses (Glover and O'Connor 2002). New evidence from South Asia has implicated maternal depression in failure to thrive, particularly at age six months, and the risk of malnutrition (Rahman *et al.* 2004; Baker-Henningham *et al.* 2003; Patel *et al.* 2003).

Maternal risk-taking behaviour during pregnancy is also thought to be more likely in the presence of depression (Milberger *et al.* 1996). Implicated in poor clinic attendance, maternal depression also appears to be predictive of low birthweight and preterm delivery (Hedegaard *et al.* 1993; Pagel *et al.* 1990; Cooper *et al.* 1996).

Midwives have an important role in the detection, prevention and support in perinatal depression. Women share an intimate relationship that is unique; this may be used to great advantage for the whole family. Failure to do this places women's mental health, family health and relationships at risk. There may be relationship breakdowns, failure to return to work, social and financial problems, avoidance of health screening and the unseen impact of health in the longer term.

Midwives work in multidisciplinary teams in providing holistic care; this will be further supported with the emergence of children's centres building upon the success of the Sure Start principles. This can only ensure that women are at the centre of that care and highlight their health as integral to the health and future of their family.

Conclusion

There is no doubt that women's mental health is emerging as a serious public health phenomenon, this fact is not just attributable to the UK but as a global concern (WHO 2000). The monetary cost to the world health economy is incalculable, but the future of generations to come rests upon timely interventions and understanding the issues surrounding this illness.

There is overwhelming evidence, through maternal death reporting in the UK, that women are at greater risk of developing a mental illness during the childbirth period than at any other time in their lives. This risk includes suicide. Both issues in turn adversely affect children and families, sometimes for their foreseeable future.

Midwives must make themselves accessible to women and aim to be the first point of contact during pregnancy, providing both a window of opportunity for identification of risk, enhancement of mental well-being and continued support for the duration of the childbearing period. It may mean working in close collaboration with other health professionals to provide specialist care, and acting as a supporter and advocate for women – which is what midwives do best. As services change to accommodate new policies and embrace current evidence, it is vital that women's and midwives voices are heard together.

Key implications for midwifery practice

- Ensure women and families have local access to information about maternal health.
- Engage all stakeholders: GPs, midwives, HV, Practice nurses, local pharmacies, nursery nurses, sexual health services, common mental health teams, voluntary services, mental health advocacy, social services, the wider community, etc.
- Promote local and national self-help groups to support women e.g. websites, complementary therapy services.

References

American Psychiatric Association (1994) *Diagnostic and Statistical Manual of Mental Disorders* (DSM IV) (4th ed). Washington, DC, American Psychiatric Association.

Angermeyer M, Matschinger H (2005) The stigma of mental illness in Germany: a trends analysis. *International Journal of Social Psychiatry* 51(3): 276–84.

Appleby L (1991) Suicide during pregnancy and in the first postnatal year. *British Medical Journal* 302: 137–40.

Appleby L, Warner R, Whitters A *et al.* (1997) A controlled study of fluoxe-
tine and cognitive-behavioural counselling in the treatment of postnatal
depression. *British Medical Journal* 314(7085): 932–36.

Association of Postnatal Illness website: www.apni.org/ (accessed
5/12/06).

Astbury J (1996) *Crazy For You: The Making of Women's Madness.*
Melbourne, Oxford University Press.

Austin MP (2004) Antenatal screening and early intervention for 'perinatal' distress, depression and anxiety: where to from here? *Archives of
Women's Mental Health* 7(1): 1–6.

Baker-Henningham H, Powell C, Walker S *et al.* (2003) Mothers of undernourished Jamaican children have poorer psychosocial functioning and
this is associated with stimulation provided in the home. *European
Journal of Clinical Nutrition* 57(6): 786–92.

Bambauer K, Prigerson H (2006) The stigma receptivity scale and its association with mental health service use among bereaved older adults.
Journal of Nervous and Mental Disorders 194(2) 139–41.

Barney L, Griffiths K, Jorm A *et al.* (2006) Stigma about depression and its
impact on help-seeking intentions. *Australian and New Zealand Journal of
Psychiatry* 40(1): 51–54.

Beck C (2004) Birth trauma is in the eye of the beholder. *Nursing Research*
53: 1.

Beech B, Robinson J (1985) Nightmares following childbirth. *British
Journal of Psychiatry* 147: 586.

Bindman J, Johnson S, Szmucker G *et al.* (2000) Continuity of care and
clinical outcome: a prospective cohort study. *Social Psychiatry and
Psychiatric Epidemiology* 35(6): 242–48.

Birth Trauma Association website: www.birthtraumaassociation.org.uk/
(accessed 5/12/06).

Brockington I (1996) *Maternal Mental Health.* Oxford, Oxford University
Press.

Campbell S, Cohn J, Meyers T (1995) Depression in first-time mothers:
mother–infant interaction and depression chronicity. *Developmental
Psychology* 31(3): 349–57.

Campbell S, Cohn J. (1996) The timing and chronicity of postpartum
depression: implications in infant development. In Murray L, Cooper PJ
(eds) *Postpartum Depression and Child Development.* New York, Guilford
Press.

Caplan H, Cogill S, Alexandra H *et al.* (1989) Maternal depression and the
emotional development of the child. *British Journal of Psychiatry* 154:
818–823.

Confidential Enquiry into Maternal and Child Health (CEMACH) (2004)
Why Mothers Die 2000–2002. London, RCOG Press.

Church S, Scanlan M (2002) Meeting the needs of women with mental
health problems. The role of the midwife in perinatal mental health
services. *The Practising Midwife* 5(5): 10–12.

Cogill S, Caplan H, Alexandra H *et al.* (1986) Impact of postnatal depression on cognitive development in young children. *British Medical Journal* 192(6529): 1165–67.

Cohn J, Matias R, Tronick E *et al.* (1986) Face-to-face interactions of depressed mothers and their infants. In Tronick E, Field T (eds) *Maternal Depression and Infant Disturbance.* San Francisco, CA, Jossey Bass, pp 31–45.

Cooper R, Goldenberg R, Das A *et al.* (1996) The preterm prediction study: maternal stress is associated with spontaneous preterm birth at less than thirty-five weeks gestation. *American Journal of Obstetrics and Gynecology* 175(5): 1286–92.

Cox JL, Connor Y, Kendall RE (1982) Prospective study of the psychiatric disorders of childbirth. *British Journal of Psychiatry* (140): 111–17.

Cox JL (1988) Causes and consequences: the life event of childbirth: sociocultural aspects of postnatal depression. In Kumar R, Brockington IF (eds) *Motherhood and Mental Illness*, vol 2. London, Butterworths, pp 64–77.

Cox JL, Holden J, Sagovsky R (1987) Detection of postnatal depression. Development of the 10-item Edinburgh Postnatal Depression Scale. *British Journal of Psychiatry* 150: 782–86.

Cox JL, Murray D, Chapman G (1993) A controlled study of onset, duration and prevalence of postnatal depression. *British Journal of Psychiatry* (163): 27–31.

Currid TJ (2004) Improving perinatal mental health care. *The Practising Midwife* 19(3): 40–43.

Cutrona C, Troutman B (1986) Social support, infant temperament, and parenting self-efficacy: a mediational model of postpartum depression. *Child Development* 57(6): 1507–18.

Das A, Olfson M, McCurtis H *et al.* (2006) Depression in African Americans: breaking barriers to detection and treatment. *Journal of Family Practice* 55(1): 30–39.

De Tychey C, Spitz E, Briancon S *et al.* (2005) Pre- and postnatal depression and coping: a comparative approach. *Journal of Affective Disorders* 85(3): 323–26.

DeMott K, Bick D, Norman R *et al.* (2006) *Clinical Guidelines and Evidence Review for Postnatal care: Routine postnatal care of recently delivered women and their babies.* London, National Collaborating Centre for Primary Care and Royal College of General Practitioners.

Department for Education and Skills (2003) *Every Child Matters: Change for Children.* London, The Stationery Office. www.dfes.gov.uk/everychildmatters/ (accessed 4/12/06).

Department of Health (1998) *Why Mothers Die. Report on Confidential Enquiries into Maternal Deaths in the United Kingdom (1994–1996).* London, The Stationery Office.

Department of Health (1999) *National Service Framework for Mental Health: Modern Standards and Service Models for Mental Health.* London, The Stationery Office.

Department of Health (2000) *The NHS plan. A Plan For Investment, a Plan for Reform*. London, The Stationery Office.

Department of Health (2002) *Women's Mental Health: Into the Mainstream*. London, The Stationery Office.

Department of Health (2003) *Women's Mental Health: Into the Mainstream, Analysis of responses to the consultation document*. London, The Stationery Office.

Department of Health (2004) *National Service Framework for children, young people and maternity services*. London, The Stationery Office.

Douglas J, Arias T (2002) *Mental Health. Midwives in Action: a resource*. London, ENB.

Evans J, Heron J, Oke S, Golding J (2001) Cohort study of depressed mood during pregnancy and after childbirth. *British Medical Journal* (323): 257–60.

Field T (1984) Early interactions between infants and their postpartum depressed mothers. *Infant Behaviour and Development* 7(4): 517–22.

Field T, Sandberg D, Garcia R *et al.* (1985) Pregnancy problems, postpartum depression and early mother–infant interactions. *Developmental Psychology* 21(6): 1152–56.

Field T, Healy B, Goldstein S *et al.* (1988) Infants of depressed mothers show 'depressed' behaviour even with non-depressed adults. *Child Development* 59(6): 1569–79.

Forman DN, Videbech P, Hedegaard MD, Salvig JD, Sechner NJ (2000) Postpartum depression: identification of women at risk. *British Journal of Obstetrics and Gynaecology* 107: 1210–17.

Gary FA (2005) Stigma: barrier to mental health care among ethnic minorities. *Issues with Mental Health Nursing* 26(10): 979–99.

Gavin N, Gaynes B, Lohr K *et al.* (2004) Perinatal depression, a systematic review: prevalence and incidence. *Obstetrics and Gynaecology* 106(1): 1071–83.

Ghodsian M, Zajicek E, Wolkind S (1984) A longitudinal study of maternal depression and child behaviour problems. *Child Psychiatry and Human Development* 25(1): 165–181.

Glover V, O'Connor T (2002) Effects of antenatal distress and anxiety: implications for development and psychiatry. *British Journal of Psychiatry* 180: 389–91.

Gutteridge K (2002) Postnatal depression: an integrative psychotherapeutic group approach. *MIDIRS Midwifery Digest* 12: 85–88.

Halbreich U (2005) The association between pregnancy process, preterm delivery, low birth weight and postnatal depression: the need for interdisciplinary integration. *American Journal of Obstetrics and Gynecology* 193(4): 1312–22.

Hanley J (1998) Postnatal depression. *Nursing Management* 4(8): 12–13.

Hart A, Lockey R, Henwood F *et al.* (2001) *Addressing Inequalities in Health: new directions in midwifery education and practice*. Research report service No 20. London, ENB.

Hay D, Kumar R (1995) Interpreting the effects of mothers' postnatal depression on children's intelligence: a critique and reanalysis. *Child Psychiatry and Human Development* 25(3): 165–81.

Hay D, Pawlby S, Sharp D *et al.* (2001) Intellectual problems shown by 11-year-old children whose mothers had postnatal depression. *Journal of Child Psychology and Psychiatry* 42(7): 871–89.

Hearn G, Illiff A, Jones I *et al.* (1998) Postnatal depression in the community. *British Journal of General Practice* 48(428): 1064–66.

Hedegaard M, Henriksen T, Sabroe S *et al.* (1993) Psychological distress in pregnancy and preterm delivery. *British Medical Journal* 307(6898): 234–39.

Kendell RE, Chalmers J, Platz C (1987) Epidemiology of puerperal psychosis. *British Journal of Psychiatry* 150: 662–673.

Kumar R, Marks M, Jackson K (1995) Prevention and treatment of postnatal psychiatric disorders. *British Journal of Midwifery* 3(6): 314–17.

Lyons-Ruth K, Zoll D, Connell D *et al.* (1986) The depressed mother and her one-year-old infant: environment, interaction, attachment and infant development. In Tronick E, Field T (eds) *Maternal Depression and Infant Disturbance.* San Francisco, CA, Jossey Bass.

Mastroianni AC, Faden R, Federman S (1994) *Women and Health Research: ethical and legal issues of including women in clinical studies.* Washington DC, Institute of Medicine, National Academy Press.

Milberger S, Biederman J, Farone S *et al.* (1996) Is maternal smoking during pregnancy a risk factor for attention deficit hyperactivity disorder in children? *American Journal of Psychiatry* 153(9): 1138–42.

Murray L (1992) The impact of postnatal depression on infant development. *Journal of Child Psychology and Psychiatry* 33(3): 543–61.

Murray L, Fiori-Cowley A, Hooper R (1996) The impact of postnatal depression and associated adversity on early mother–infant interactions and later infant outcome. *Child Development* 67(5): 2512–16.

Murray L, Hipwell A, Hooper R *et al.* (1996) The cognitive development of 5-year-old children of postnatally depressed mothers. *Journal of Child Psychology and Psychiatry* 37(8): 927–36.

Murray JL, Lopez AD (1996a) *The Global Burden of Disease: A comprehensive assessment of mortality and disability from diseases, injuries and risk factors in 1990 and projected to 2020.* Summary. Boston: Harvard School of Public Health, World Health Organization.

Murray CJ, Lopez AD (1996b) Evidence-based health policy: lessons from the Global Burden of Disease Study. *Science* 274: 740–43.

National Institute for Clinical Excellence (2005) *Post-traumatic Stress Disorder (PTSD): The management of PTSD in adults and children in primary and secondary care.* London, NICE Publications.

Nursing and Midwifery Council (2004) *Midwives Rules and Standards.* London, NMC.

Oates M (1994) *Postnatal Mental Illness: organisation and function of services in perinatal psychiatry.* London, Gaskell Press, pp 8–33.

Oates M (2000) *Perinatal Mental Health Services*. London, The Royal College of Psychiatrists.

Oates M (2001) Deaths from psychiatric causes. In *Why Mothers Die. The fifth report of the Confidential Enquiry into Maternal deaths in the United Kingdom (1997–1999)* London, RCOG pp 165–87.

Olde E, van der Hart O, Kleber R, van Son M (2006) Post-traumatic stress following childbirth: a review. *Clinical Psychology Review* 26(1): 1–16.

Pagel M, Smilkstein G, Regen H *et al.* (1990) Psychosocial influences on newborn outcomes: a controlled perspective study. *Social Science and Medicine* 30(5): 597–604.

Parkes S, Hardy B (1997) Postnatal depression: making better use of health visitors and CPNs. *Professional Care of Mother and Child* 7(6): 151–52.

Patel V, De Sousa N, Rodrigues M (2003) Postnatal depression and infant growth and development in low-income countries: a cohort study from Goa, India. *Archives of Diseases in Childhood* 88(1): 34–37.

Rahman A, Lovel H, Bunn J *et al.* (2004) Mothers' mental health and infant growth: a case-control study from Rawalpindi, Pakistan. *Child Care and Health Development* 30(1): 21–27.

Raphael-Leff J (2001) *Psychological Processes of Childbearing* (revised edition) CPS Psychoanalytical Publication Series, University of Essex.

Ritterford V, Jin S (2006) Addressing media stigma of people experiencing mental illness using an entertainment–education strategy. *Journal of Health Psychology* 11(2): 247–67.

Robinson J, Beech B (1991) Suicide in pregnancy. *British Medical Journal* 302: 5912.

Robinson J (1998) Suicide: a major cause of maternal deaths. *British Journal of Midwifery* 6(12): 167.

Ross-Davie M, Elliot S, Sarkar A, Green L (2006) A public health role in perinatal mental health: are midwives ready? *British Journal of Midwifery* 14(6): 330–34.

Royal College of Obstetricians and Gynaecologists (2001) *Why Mothers Die: Confidential Enquiries into Maternal Deaths (1997–1999)* London, RCOG.

Royal College of Psychiatrists (2000) *Perinatal Maternal Mental Health Services*. Council Report CR88. London, Royal College of Psychiatrists.

Ryding E, Wijma K, Wijma B (1998) Predisposing psychological factors for post-traumatic stress reactions after emergency caesarean section. *Acta Obstetricia et Gynecologica Scandinavica* 77: 351–52.

Saltman D (1991) *Women and Health: an introduction*. Sydney, Harcourt Brace Jovanovich.

Shakespeare J (2001) *Evaluation of screening for postnatal depression against the NCS handbook criteria*. UK, National Screening Committee.

Sharp D, Hay D, Pawlby S *et al.* (1995) The impact of postnatal depression on boys' intellectual development. *Journal of Child Psychology and Psychiatry* 36(8): 1315–37.

Sinclair D, Murray L (1998) Effects of postnatal depression on children's adjustment to school: teachers' reports. *British Journal of Psychiatry* 172: 58–63.

Small R, Lumley J, Donohue L *et al.* (2000) Randomised controlled trial of midwife-led debriefing to reduce maternal depression after operative childbirth. *British Medical Journal* 321: 1043–47.

Small R, Lumley J, Toomey L (2006) Midwife-led debriefing after operative birth: four to six year follow-up of a randomised trial. *BMC Medicine* 4: 3.

Spitzer R, Endicott J, Robins E (1978) Research diagnostic criteria: rationale and reliability. *Archives of General Psychiatry* 35(7): 773–82.

Stewart C, Henshaw C (2002) Midwives and perinatal mental health. *British Journal of Midwifery* 10(2): 117–21.

Stuart H (2006) Media portrayal of mental illness and its treatments: What effect does it have on people with mental illness? *CNS Drugs* 20(2): 99–106.

Thoppil J, Riutcel T, Nalesnik S *et al.* (2005) Early intervention for perinatal depression. *American Journal of Obstetrics and Gynecology* 192(5): 1446–48.

Tully L, Garcia J, Davidson L, Marchant S (2002) Role of midwives in depression screening. *British Journal of Midwifery* 10(6): 374–78.

Van Dorn R, Swanson J, Elbogen E *et al.* (2005) A comparison of stigmatising attitudes toward persons with schizophrenia in four stakeholder groups: perceived likelihood of violence and desire for social distance. *Psychiatry* 68(2): 152–163.

Watson JP, Elliott SA, Rugg AJ, Brough DI (1984) Psychiatric disorder in pregnancy and the first postnatal year. *British Journal of Psychiatry* 144: 453–462.

Whiffen V (1991) The comparison of postpartum with non-postpartum depression: a rose by any other name. *J Psychiatry Neuroscience.* September 16(3): 160–165.

Whiffen V, Gotlib I (1989) Infants of postpartum depressed mother: temperament and cognitive status. *Journal of Abnormal Psychology* 98(3): 274–79.

Wieck A, Kumar R, Hurst A *et al.* (1991) Increased sensitivity of dopamine receptors and recurrence of affective psychosis after childbirth. *British Medical Journal* 303(6813): 613–16.

Wilson LM, Reid AJ, Midmer DK *et al.* (1996) Antenatal psychosocial risk factors associated with adverse postnatal family outcomes. *Canadian Medical Association* (154): 785–99.

World Health Organization (WHO) (1992) *International Classification of Disease: 10 (ICD-10).* Geneva, World Health Organization.

World Health Organization (WHO) (2000) *Women's Mental Health: An Evidence Based Review.* Geneva, World Health Organization.

Wrate R, Rooney A, Thomas P *et al.* (1985) Postnatal depression and child development: a three-year follow-up study. *British Journal of Psychiatry* 146: 622–27.

Chapter 9
Supporting Breastfeeding: Midwives Facilitating a Community Model

*Sue Henry, Fiona Dykes, Sheena Byrom, Michelle Atkin
and Elaine Jackson*

> Breastfeeding is a natural 'safety net' against the worst effects
> of poverty . . . exclusive breastfeeding goes a long way toward
> cancelling out the health difference between being born into
> poverty and being born into affluence . . . It is almost as if
> breastfeeding takes the infant out of poverty for those first few
> months in order to give the child a fairer start in life and com-
> pensate for the injustice of the world into which it was born
> (James P Grant, former Executive Director, UNICEF)

The baby feeding culture

Breastfeeding has become a major public health issue. In the UK,
for example, in 2000, 85% of mothers in higher socioeconomic
occupational groups commenced breastfeeding compared with
59% in lower socioeconomic occupational groups, as defined by
the national statistics socioeconomic classification (Hamlyn *et al.*
2002). There is a similar inequity in duration rates of breastfeeding
with 75% of women who commence breastfeeding in higher socioeconomic occupational groups still breastfeeding at six weeks, but
only 53% of women who commence breastfeeding in lower socioeconomic occupational groups continuing at six weeks (Hamlyn
et al. 2002).

This inequity from birth constitutes a crucial aspect of the transmitted cycle of nutritional deprivation (Barker 1994; Dykes and
Hall Moran 2006) and it is now recognised that two of the government priority areas for health improvement, coronary health
and cancer reduction could be positively impacted by increasing

breastfeeding rates (DoH 2000). The inequity with regard to infant feeding method was highlighted in the government's NHS Plan in which a commitment to increase breastfeeding rates by 2004 formed part of the proposed strategy to improve diet and nutrition (DoH 2000). In line with the government position, the Maternity Care Working Party (2001) document *Modernising Maternity Care: A Commissioning Toolkit for Primary Care Trusts in England* advocated that service providers should demonstrate effective breastfeeding policies and practices that ensured ongoing support to breastfeeding mothers. Further commitment to increasing breastfeeding rates was reflected in *Improvement, Expansion and Reform: The Next Three Years Priorities and Planning Framework 2003–2006* (DoH 2002). The momentum for promotion of breastfeeding continues with the recent publication of two further public health documents *Choosing Health* (DoH 2005a) and *Choosing a Better Diet* (DoH 2005b). Again these documents emphasise the connections between socioeconomic deprivation and suboptimal diet and infant feeding practices.

Strategies to support women to breastfeed

In their evidence into practice briefing, Dyson and colleagues (2006) cite as some of the reasons for low breastfeeding rates in the UK:

- Societal and cultural influences
- Poor continuity of care in health services
- Clinical problems
- Lack of preparation of health professionals and others to support breastfeeding effectively.

The document states that women may be influenced positively or negatively by the experiences of their family and friends, media messages and advice from midwife or GP. Because health services now have this invaluable resource, which identifies significant barriers to breastfeeding, local and national strategies may be developed to support women in their decision to breastfeed their baby. Dyson and colleagues (2006) outline nine recommendations for organisations to implement, which have the potential to increase initiation and continuation of breastfeeding rates. One of the proposals is for hospital and community NHS services providers to implement the United Nationals Children's Fund (UNICEF) UK Baby Friendly Initiative (BFI). The BFI programme provides a framework for the implementation of best practice by NHS Trusts, other healthcare facilities and higher education institutions, with the aim of ensuring that all parents are helped to make informed decisions about feeding their babies and that they are then supported in their chosen feeding method. This recommendation is reinforced by the recent *Postnatal Care Guideline* published by the National Institute for Clinical Excellence (DeMott *et al.* 2006), which strengthens the importance of secondary and primary care services to implement an externally evaluated programme such as the BFI as a minimum standard.

By implementing the BFI within healthcare services, many of the Dyson *et al.* (2006) recommendations would be fulfilled. Effective interventions are multifaceted, and include professional and peer support (Dyson *et al.* 2006). Midwives make up a significant proportion of the professional support available to women. In a recent survey of mothers in the UK, the National Childbirth Trust (NCT) (Dodds 2006) revealed that compared with other health professionals, midwives provided new mothers with the most information about breastfeeding (77%). However, Dykes (2005a, 2006) demonstrates how 'hospital' midwives are sometimes inhibited in their quest to support women to breastfed due to organisational culture in postnatal wards. Schmied, Sheehan and Barclay (2001) propose the assumption that midwives believe they are the owners of the wisdom and knowledge necessary to breastfeed, and that this knowledge is not only authentic but paramount. This can be problematic, as breastfeeding is not a medical intervention or professionally 'owned' skill, but a social interaction between mother and baby.

Mothers supporting mothers: back to the community

In many communities in the UK, most specifically those with high levels of social deprivation, breastfeeding is often perceived and experienced as a marginal and indeed liminal activity, rarely seen and barely spoken about (Hoddinott and Pill 1999; Dykes 2003; Scott and Mostyn 2003; Sachs 2005). Women in such communities tend to lack confidence in their ability to breastfeed (Dykes and Williams 1999; Hoddinott and Pill 1999; Hawkins and Heard 2001; Dykes 2002, 2003, 2005b, 2006). Changing local cultures favourably towards breastfeeding is a necessarily slow process if sustainable changes in the prevalence and duration of breastfeeding are to be made. The implementation of community peer support schemes is being increasingly recognised as one of the key ways in which this cultural change can be achieved (Dykes 2003, 2005c; Dyson *et al.* 2006). Peer support is defined by Dennis (2003) as:

> The provision of emotional, appraisal, and informational assistance by a created social network member who possesses experiential knowledge of a specific behaviour or stressor and similar characteristics as the target population
>
> (Dennis 2003:329)

Peer supporters are positive role models for women with regard to breastfeeding (Hoddinott and Pill 1999; McInnes and Stone 2000; Anderson and Grant 2001; Alexander *et al.* 2003; Kirkham *et al.* 2006). As women are supported effectively with breast-feeding and therefore continue for longer, breastfeeding becomes more visible and others are more likely to initiate breastfeeding due to exposure to positive role models. The potential of peer support programmes to empower those living in socially excluded communities should not be underestimated (Dykes 2003, 2005c).

A number of peer support programmes have been described in the UK (Wright 1996; McInnes *et al.* 2000; Anderson and Grant 2001; Battersby 2001a,b; McInnes and Stone 2001; Battersby and Sabin 2002; Sookhoo *et al.* 2002; Timms 2002; Alexander *et al.* 2003; Dykes 2003; Raine and Woodward 2003; Scott and Mostyn 2003; Smale 2004; Kirkham *et al.* 2006) and internationally (Kistin *et al.* 1994; Long *et al.* 1995; Arlotti *et al.* 1998; Schafer *et al.* 1998; Morrow *et al.* 1999; Shaw and Kaczorowski 1999; Dennis 2002; Dennis *et al.* 2002; Haider *et al.* 2002). Dykes (2003, 2005c) in a synthesis of 26 government-funded peer-support projects described aspects that appear to be crucial to successful implementation and sustainability:

- Cultural awareness and sensitivity facilitated by local cultural assessment and in-depth understanding of the local culture, as described by others (Wright *et al.* 1997; Sellen 2001)
- Building on existing infrastructure – becoming aware of existing schemes and projects in surrounding areas and developing interconnected projects that support each other through shared experiences and in some cases personnel
- Comprehensive planning with involvement of key stakeholders in the strategic planning of change with effective communication lying at the heart of this process
- Effective systems for recruitment, selection, training and ongoing support for the peer supporters

- Peer-professional partnership – effective development and maintenance of positive relationships between peer supporters and health professionals
- An ongoing, comprehensive publicity strategy. This is crucial to community receptivity regarding the innovation and for effective uptake of the peer support schemes
- Supportive infrastructure to maintain and sustain the peer support schemes to include careful planning of referral strategies and access points
- Support group/'drop-in' centres as a focal point at which peer supporters, health professionals and breastfeeding women may meet
- Comprehensive evaluation using a robust methodology that involves a continual cycle of evaluation and subsequent implementation of improvements
- Obtaining and maintaining sustainable sources of funding.

These key elements of success may be achieved through a variety of models, some being voluntary organisation-led, some health professional-led and others peer supporter co-ordinated. In this paper we describe the development and ongoing progress of a project in the UK, that clearly fits into these aspects, Little Angels (Darwen) Ltd.

Little Angels: a breastfeeding community business

Little Angels is a mother-to-mother breastfeeding support programme that offers individual face-to-face and telephone contact to all breastfeeding mothers in a large industrial borough in East Lancashire. The service adds value to current health professional strategy to support, facilitate and empower mothers to initiate breastfeeding and to promote the continuation rate for at least six months. Little Angels contributes to the provision of a quality seamless service, for the promotion and protection of successful breastfeeding throughout the continuum of pregnancy, childbirth and early childhood through effective partnership working.

The project has evolved and expanded, and improved initiation and duration breastfeeding rates. The peer (mother) supporters are paid workers, with funding secured from various sources described below. Little Angels has limited company status, and is supported by a board that guides the business processes and decisions. Some board members have advisory roles only and as such serve the project by using their combined vast experience in health, to provide detailed and specific guidance on breastfeeding matters. Other members share their business and management experience, provide day-to-day advice, and contribute to the smooth running of the project. Little Angels employ a midwife, who is also the infant feeding coordinator from the local maternity unit, on a part-time basis. It could be suggested that this is a real example of community empowerment, with mothers employing health professionals!

How did Little Angels begin?

Michelle was expecting her fifth baby. She was sitting in a community antenatal clinic when the Sure Start midwife began to chat to her. The midwife had been around when Michelle had her previous baby, and knew she had breastfed most of her children. The midwife was also aware that Michelle was passionate about breastfeeding, and asked her if she would help set up a breastfeeding support group. Approximately eight mothers attended the first meeting, but Michelle left feeling discouraged and despondent, as she felt 'she was the only person that actually enjoyed breastfeeding'. The mothers had described their problems and how difficult breastfeeding had been for them, which had surprised Michelle, as she expected them to say how brilliant it was. Despite the group not meeting her expectations she carried on going.

The group met in a local church every two weeks, and often it was just Michelle, the Sure Start midwife and a team midwife. Then the group moved to a new building, now a children's centre, and things started to improve. It was there that Elaine sought breastfeeding support for herself and experienced what is was like to receive peer support. She soon became involved in running the group, which was increasing in popularity, and the breastfeeding rates in the area started to increase. Michelle and Elaine began providing peer support on a voluntary basis, and other mothers became interested too. They completed a local two-day course in breastfeeding management, facilitated by the maternity unit's infant feeding coordinator, and a health visitor colleague. Flowers were presented to celebrate their success.

Michelle took part in some additional training in relation to self-esteem and motivation. On completion, she made a decision to pursue her dream to earn a living supporting women to breastfeed successfully. She was, however, unsure of how that was possible – she believed that this type of work was for professional people who were medically qualified, and she was not. But the course leader encouraged her to 'create the job', and because Michelle was able to reflect on how successful the support group had been, she felt enthused. She began to provide one-to-one support in mothers' homes, going to see them for extra support for the midwives.

Michelle already worked 10 hours a week for the Sure Start local programme in addition to some voluntary work with the council. Her role in the council related to the empowerment of communities, and links there led to a discussion with colleagues about her idea to form a community business to support breastfeeding. She was given a number to ring – a local small business support company (Bootstrap). From there, she met someone who believed in her, and did not say her idea was impossible. This person gave Michelle a list of questions to do some research, and to find more people who were supportive. She discussed it with another local breastfeeding mother, who approved, but they took no action until 12 months later, when they chatted with mothers at the group about what would be 'ideal support', and what was missing from their experiences.

Elaine and Michelle were united in their excitement, and they used their renewed energy to develop their first bid together for Sure Start funding, with an aim to provide breastfeeding telephone and peer support. Together with three other interested mothers, they completed a six-week business course, which enabled them to plan their vision. Participating in the programme highlighted the fact that there were two natural leaders who were going to drive things forward. Senior personnel in the local maternity services were supportive and displayed confidence in the idea. This was important to the mothers, as they wanted to maintain strong links with the service. Then the news came; their Sure Start bid was successful, within four programmes! And that was only the beginning . . .

In 2004, this community mothers' project collaborated with the local acute (maternity services) and primary care trusts, to apply for public service agreement (PSA) funding to stretch local breastfeeding targets (see Chapter 1 for further details of PSA targets). The aim of the initiative was to promote and support the initiation of breastfeeding and to increase and sustain breastfeeding duration rates above and beyond the set 2% target at 6–8 weeks and 7–9 months, with a focus on those mothers less likely to breastfeed. The bid was successful, and the funding provided financial backing for the community business to organise, facilitate and carry out one-to-one support to breastfeeding mothers across the borough.

The objectives of the project were to:

- Ascertain areas of need in borough for enhanced support in client group
- Increase input of peer breastfeeding support on the antenatal and postnatal wards at the local maternity unit
- Promote breastfeeding in antenatal clinics in both hospital and community settings
- Offer home visits to all mothers in the area who are discharged from hospital breastfeeding
- Provide 24/7 telephone support to offer advice and help on breastfeeding issues
- Empower parents with accurate, researched information to provide needed support in a family setting
- Support and encourage family members (e.g. fathers and grandparents) so that they can help breastfeeding mothers
- Maintain or set up breastfeeding support groups
- Offer outreach support at baby clinics
- Receive and act on referrals from all health or social care workers
- Assist with and support Sure Start local programmes to become UNICEF Baby Friendly accredited
- Recruit volunteers as peer support workers and provide breast-feeding counsellor training for volunteers
- Work with the local community to promote and raise aware-ness of breastfeeding
- Liaise with local businesses to raise awareness of the rights of breastfeeding mothers returning to work and the benefit to the company
- Promote self-esteem and confidence in women to continue breastfeeding for at least six months
- Assist with dissemination of information to address common issues associated with breastfeeding, e.g. growth spurts; mast-itis; weaning
- Visit local schools to promote breastfeeding.

Support offered by the project is an 'opt-out' rather than 'opt-in' referral system. A peer supporter contacts all women who are discharged from the maternity unit within 48 hours, with the offer of one-to-one contact. Following informed consent, a visit to their home is then arranged. Practical support is combined with emo-tional support, and new mothers are encouraged to help each other. All breastfeeding support workers receive Baby Friendly Initiative, child protection and communication skills training and

updates. The team engages with volunteers who help to achieve
the objectives and are then in a position to apply for a vacant paid
position should one become available.

In the project there is an overarching aim of building capability
in local communities to promote and protect breastfeeding as
the normal and most beneficial method of infant feeding. This
service to local women and the wider community was initiated
from mothers in the same situation themselves, identifying gaps
in breastfeeding support locally. Little Angels was created by
mothers and is run successfully by mothers. The benefits of
this model are many, but two are particularly significant. In the
first instance, breastfeeding duration rates are encouraging
(Figure 9.1).

Second, the initiative reflects a community development model;
strengthening the ability of the community, building on skills,
defining and achieving objectives, managing a community project and taking part in partnerships (HDA 2004). Little Angels
represents a resource in differing sub-communities and growing
social capital is evident, as communities strengthen in their sense
of belonging and co-operation, and attitudes to breastfeeding
become more positive by engaging diverse populations from each
locality in the borough. Their activity aims to strengthen cohesion,

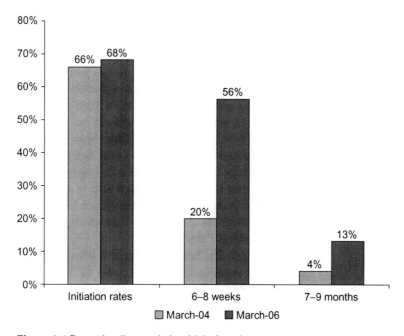

Figure 9.1 Breastfeeding statistics: Little Angels peer support.

and social engagement provides a sense of belonging. The support is becoming 'rooted' in communities, with an increasing number of members of those communities becoming aware of the work of Little Angels. Local participation in various other groups is encouraged – voluntary and professional, social and purposeful, religious and political.

The peer supporters do not view the work as a job, but a 'way of life'. The project reaches out not only to the paid workers but also to volunteers who could be family, friends, grandparents and other community neighbours. The influence of the support is owned by the community, which facilitates trust, friendships and health improvement strategies to flourish through the theme of breastfeeding support and promotion. For some supporters, it is their first paid work in the UK; they enjoy working with mothers from their local community, creating special bonds and relationships. Their contribution to this chapter was sought, and is described below.

Influencing change: shifting 'cultures'

The peer supporters shared their experiences and feelings about what breastfeeding means to them, and how working closely with mothers had influenced their thoughts and beliefs. Trudy described how she would previously have frowned upon people who did not breastfeed, but with her experience now she could look at women 'as a whole and understand better what influences their decisions'. She feels she is not as judgmental. Miriam commented how her experiences as a supporter had changed how she feels about breastfeeding. She came from a culture where it was expected that she would breastfeed, so she never previously considered anything different. Her own two babies presented her with different experiences – one negative and one positive. Farzana had not breastfed her own children – it did not feel natural or comfortable for her. Now that she is supporting mothers to breastfeed, she would like the experience for herself. She feels that supporting mothers to breastfeed has changed her whole view and she 'feels fantastic' about it.

Jane formula fed her first baby and breastfed her second. After this second experience she felt 'part of the breastfeeding club' and was meeting new mothers. So not only enjoying the health benefits, Jane is also experiencing the social benefits of breastfeeding. Jane feels she now has the strength to say she understands the difference between breast and bottlefeeding, because she has had two different experiences. Some of the supporters view breast milk as a gift, 'the best gift a mother can give to her baby'. Anne shared her thoughts describing how she felt that breastfeeding is the future of our children, educating them, building them up to know about breastfeeding, about the health benefits. She enjoys giving information to mothers in hospital and being a part of their decision on how to feed their baby. Anne described how she talks to mothers who formula feed their baby too, giving them information. She also enjoys giving information in schools, and watching her own daughter breastfeed her doll, hoping she in turn will tell her own children one day. Paula believes breastfeeding to be the 'ultimate experience', agreeing it 'can be tough at first', and to be able to empower mothers and help them through it is the 'biggest buzz ever'. Anne described how women will often say, 'I can't do this', and then the supporter says, 'come on, keep trying' and weeks later they are still breastfeeding – 'I know my work is valuable then'. 'The women succeed themselves, and this is the ultimate in job satisfaction, to sit back, see and smile.'

Celebrating diversity; learning from others

Employing peer supporters from the very heart of local communities has many hidden advantages. Parveen laughed as she revealed her age of 45, and explains why she feels this is an advantage as mothers in South Asian communities address her as 'Auntie' and welcome her so much. Parveen described her joy when she meets mothers at the local school gates and they tell her 'I'm still breastfeeding!' She responds cheekily to them, 'Good, if you stop, I won't visit you!' This direct approach, which works well in Parveen's community and is respected by all, would not perhaps be acceptable in other cultures. Parveen visited one mother 21 times in one week, made possible due to the close proximity to her home and the close relationships that had developed. The mother called the supporter her 'second mum'. Understanding community issues is crucial, and language barriers can sometimes be problematic. Employing staff from within a community helps to overcome these issues and it enhances the sharing of what works from culture to culture. Likewise, sometimes 'matching' peer supporters with mothers can help. Little Angels employs a 'young mother' to specifically work with younger new mothers. It creates that 'trendy' image which appeals to the young mothers and a sense of 'if she can do it, so can I'.

Demedicalising breastfeeding

The supporters described their desire to 'demedicalise' breastfeeding, and to bring 'it back to the mothers'. They are happy to be able to give so much time, not being rushed as health professionals sometimes are. Supporters in Little Angels feel it makes successful breastfeeding more a 'reality' when support comes from another mother and not a health professional. If a mother says 'yes you can do it and it is worthwhile' then it means so much. The women also believe that mother-led breastfeeding support groups help to encourage mothers to continue to feed for longer. Gail remembers seeing a two-year-old being breastfed and being surprised. She then herself fed her two-year-old and believed the influence to be the mother at the group. Sometimes if a supporter visits a mother from a different culture, class or age they wonder about the word 'peer', and the word 'mother' is often used. Some supporters say they prefer to work in the area where they live as they feel more 'equal' – not entering a house at a 'higher level', and they feel more 'connected'. They expressed the view that women 'sometimes take you into their home like a family member'. The supporters see mothers in the hospital and in their homes, which brings particular rewards through continuity. Many women keep contact even when they actually stop breastfeeding.

'Just being there'

The flexibility of peer support is a bonus for peer supporters, as most have young families. Teamwork is essential, they all help each other. Feedback from mothers is usually positive, many sending thank-you messages and support for Little Angels. Sonia recalls struggling with a woman for a long time with painful feeding and remembers the woman ringing her to say: 'I just want you to know the pain has gone and I wouldn't be still feeding now without your support.' It meant so much to Sonia, and although the supporters know they have not always got the answer to problems, they usually have and feel that 'just being there' has turned situations around so many times. Many mothers value the telephone contact – always somebody on the other end of the line, not a machine but a person who is available day or night. This is a voluntary part of the Little Angels work, a part they know is important to women. The supporters are delighted when they see women breastfeeding who they never would have thought would even try, and when the mothers themselves tell them that they never imagined they could.

Partnerships

Working with relevant agencies has been crucial to the ongoing success of this project. 'Bootstrap', a community organisation which supports the development and ongoing guidance of Little Angels, provides business advice and assistance with writing bids for funding. Children's centre partnerships have been challenging at times, but also very supportive, and have provided the project with opportunities to be creative in their work. Local and national telephone helplines are given to all new mothers at the local hospital, with the names and contacts for support groups. The support received through Little Angels is made available to all mothers regardless of what support they are receiving from other sources. Little Angels liaises with national support groups over current issues and seeks their advice and information at times. Relationships have been built with health professionals, and the support offered is mutual, with cross-referral systems being the key! General practitioners, paediatricians and hospital registrars have contacted them for support and advice.

Professional representation and support is available within the management structure of the project, and includes the consultant midwife and infant feeding co-ordinator from the local maternity unit, Children's Centre manager, health visitors, primary care trust (PCT) professional leads and a senior academic from the local university. The project is fortunate to sit in a borough that has unitary authority status[1], and works in tandem with the local PCT. This gives strength to the group, as there are shared targets, i.e. PSA targets, of which breastfeeding is one. The community business model, aiming to improve breastfeeding rates, fits within the objectives of the local authority, and so there is a 'win-win' situation. Little Angels works closely with policy department at the local authority, and neighbourhood renewal funding (NRF) came from the 'Extending People's Lives' strand of the budget; an example of the local commitment to breastfeeding.

Linking into mixed discipline meetings or groups helps to share good practice and formulate new ideas. A Breastfeeding Initiative Group at the maternity unit meets monthly, and Little Angels participate in the agenda. This provides an opportunity for them to liaise with midwives, health visitors, other breastfeeding supporters and professional leads. Children's centre meetings also provide relevant local contacts.

The peer supporters are involved in activities in the maternity unit, including teaching student midwives. Four Little Angels supporters deliver the two-day UNICEF breastfeeding management course along with midwives and health visitors *for* health visitors, midwives and other peer supporters! Working together with midwives in the first few weeks is an example of true partnership working; both need each other. The professionals have contacts, knowledge and experience, which are always valued and appreciated. The peer supporters have more time to devote to one subject that they are passionate about. The whole process hinges on collaborative relationships for its success, and on having a great team of likeminded people.

Ongoing personal development

All peer supporters working in Little Angels are trained in breastfeeding support, and many have completed the La Leche League peer support training. The latter provides an excellent opportunity for the workers to reflect on what peer support means, learning from each other about what mothers really need. Sharing and debriefing time is very useful, using personal experiences to reflect and progress, which helped the development of working methods, looking at strengths and assets. The training brought everyone together with one learning theme. It soon became apparent that knowledge was not the only thing needed for peer support, but unconditional time, being open about feelings, commitment and effective communication skills.

All volunteers and peer supporters attended the two-day course on breastfeeding management (based on a UNICEF modular approach) in the local maternity unit, which has maintained Baby Friendly status since 1997. They learn side-by-side with health professionals, promoting consistency of approach and methods. All breastfeeding supporters are then able to provide consistent information and teach practical skills in the same way, to maximise the mothers' confidence. In this module, the supporters are given support in developing communication skills including listening skills, suggesting rather than advising, and understanding. They gain an insight into providing true informed choice, marketing of breastmilk substitutes, in addition to how to provide support for common difficulties. Some of the workers have undertaken Breastfeeding Network training and all have had extra input from the National Childbirth Trust. Elaine and Michelle are both qualified to deliver the La Leche League peer support administrator training.

Little Angels also participate in 'in-house' workshops on subjects such as positioning and attachment, hand expression, thrush and mastitis, insufficient milk, weaning, bed sharing, re-lactation, sudden infant death syndrome and special situations. Communication skills are always revisited. Role-play affords staff the opportunity to explore different options together in a 'safe place'.

It is essential that all the breastfeeding supporters are themselves supported in their work. New supporters receive a thorough induction and a period of support as the work can be quite lonely at times. The opportunity for a lead (Elaine, Sue or Michelle) to work with a supporter is offered frequently both in the hospital and community – during home visits, antenatal clinics and support groups. All supporters are allocated to a mentor, who provides debriefing time and encouragement. The mentors (also supporters) have extra time to do this role effectively. 'Care for carers' meetings, also facilitated by the mentor on a regular basis, help provide support. Positive and negative feedback is shared and learning and support is achieved. Supporters must be valued and feel free to discuss openly on any matter. The supporters ask for suggestions, and responses are valued. Frequent meetings – informal and formal – help with feedback from mothers and other staff disciplines. Employees in the project have formed close friendships; they provide ongoing support for each other in many ways, stemming from a deep desire to succeed.

Integration

The presence and participation of Little Angels in the hospital has been outstanding, resulting in mothers receiving high quality extra support.

Little Angels provide support on the postnatal wards, in antenatal clinics, and they facilitate a daily support group in the maternity unit for mothers. The sessions are also accessible to – and well attended by – women on the antenatal wards, who are able to gain information on positioning and attachment and hand expression. New and expectant mothers also explore how breastfeeding works, how to maximise milk production and flow, and where to get support when at home. Questions are encouraged and open informal discussions follow. The sessions provide an opportunity for women to meet and then provide ongoing support for each other after the group ends. The supporters also visit and assist mothers whose babies are on the neonatal intensive care unit, sitting with them during expressing times or early feeds, and providing emotional support.

In May 2005 the supporters integrated into midwifery teams; each team was allocated one or two 'Little Angels'. This development facilitated increased community continuity with shared support between professionals and peer supporters. Little Angels supporters always refer deviations from normal to a health professional, but their support continues until the mother stops breastfeeding, whatever that age might be.

Making breastfeeding fashionable!

Little Angels has a publicity strategy, including a website (www.littleangels.org.uk/), with the aim to promote the 'normality' of breastfeeding. They developed a poster campaign using photographs of local women. These are accompanied by catchy slogans, with the intention of getting away from the usual health benefits of breastfeeding. The rationale for this strategy was that although women know the health benefits of breastfeeding, the rates remain low. The group also developed a calendar, which was distributed freely to NHS trusts in the country.

For World Breastfeeding Week Little Angels each year organise a 'mummy milk march', to raise awareness locally. A large group of mothers, prams and babies and the local mayor always stimulates interest, and when the public ask what is happening, breastfeeding is discussed. The activity has the potential to promote confidence in mothers who choose to breastfeed – they all get together and support each other. Other events Little Angels respond to include National Breastfeeding Awareness Week and Green Week. Little Angels also featured on a Channel 4 (2006) documentary called *Extraordinary Breastfeeding*.

Michelle believes that the voice of support for breastfeeding is crucial. She approaches dignitaries including councillors to help her and has been fortunate to be in contact with many who have been willing to listen and help her. The team has regularly been invited to present their work throughout the UK, and recently in Northern Ireland.

Supporting support groups

Little Angels provide support to existing breastfeeding groups in the local communities and have invested in the development of further groups. They discovered that different communities need local, accessible support groups. One particular successful development is a group held in a local leisure centre, which is easily accessed with prams, is central to the town, and has a large space for toys and equipment. One strong advantage of this venue is the link with sport, fitness and leisure: many mothers attending after toddler swim time. For some mothers it could be an introduction to the leisure centre and its facilities such as gym/swim with crèches, aquanatal for postnatal mothers with crèche. The leisure centre café provides sandwiches and drinks for the women at a reasonable cost. A sense of well-being and meeting new friends helps a mother's emotional well-being too!

Another group has been developed by a supporter who is from South Asian heritage. Farzana is pivotal in providing the right environment and welcome for Asian mothers in her community, bringing everyone together for breastfeeding support and socialising. Lastly, there is now a support group for breastfeeding toddlers at a local central soft play facility, alongside an already established mother and tots group.

Evaluation

A robust system for collecting information on breastfeeding mothers was implemented in partnership with the research midwife co-ordinator in the local maternity unit. This data collection sheet known locally as the 'tracker' collects information on feeding method at birth, at 6 weeks, at 17 weeks, at 6 months, at 7–9 months, at 12 months and the age of weaning. It also provides details of when the first breastfeed was initiated, any use of formula, teats/dummies in hospital, the attendance at support groups, supporter contact details and the involvement of significant others. The form allows for explanation of the reason for giving up breastfeeding; and allows space for other comments. This statistical tool assists Little Angels to track what is happening locally with postcode reference, and see how and if breastfeeding rates are changing as a result of the support being provided. As mentioned previously, the results so far are encouraging (see Table 9.1). There has been funding awarded[2] to carry out a qualitative evaluation of Little Angels by studying 10 women's personal accounts of the support they received. The results from the interviews will inform the development of a questionnaire, which will be sent to a statistically calculated number of mothers who have been supported. A local mother external to the project, has been trained in basic research and interviewing skills, and she will facilitate interviews with the women.

What's good about working for Little Angels?

The individual supporters appreciate the camaraderie and friendship in the team, and enjoy working with health and social care workers. All members of the team rely on each other, and there is a strong sense of commitment. They are proud of their breastfeeding success. Family-friendly approaches are appreciated, with flexibility of hours to suit personal needs. They believe they have their ideal, perfect job and although some days are stressful and busy, all agree it is worth it. The development of 'mentors' within the supporting staff has been invaluable for their support, debriefing and reflection time. As mentioned earlier, for some peer supporters it is their first paid employment, and others have left their jobs to work for Little Angels. Everyone has changed in some way.

The supporters feel a great sense of achievement. Kauser informed us that this is her first job, her mother had a stroke and her husband had a heart attack. She was feeling depressed and then Little Angels offered her a job. Now she feels every day she is 'reborn'. She knows when she sees a baby feeding and talks to mothers in their home that she couldn't have 'done better'. Other supporters expressed their delight in the work:

- I get in my car and I know I'm going to work and the clouds are lifted
- I enjoy myself so much it isn't like a job
- You don't know who you'll meet, every day's different and it's just so rewarding and I feel honoured to be doing it
- It's a job that I could never have imagined
- I don't feel stress at work
- You forget everything . . . all that matters is that mum and baby.

The future

Little Angels would like to maximise the support they give locally and to assist and support as many mothers as possible. They have been invited to expand the project in a neighbouring borough due to the success in their local area. They want to use the evidence to support peer supporters everywhere and to influence local and national strategies.

There are some new mothers who have never seen anyone breastfeed their baby. Michelle recalled one mother who was seeking asylum in the UK coming to the support group and not being able to understand the purpose or concept of such a group. 'Breastfeeding just happens', she said. In her country breastfeeding was all she saw; mothers see and they just learn. Little Angels hope to bring this kind of breastfeeding culture to the forefront of communities through their influence and support.

Points for reflection: a mother's reflection

Sure Start has been a wonderful experience in our area and the Sure Start midwife, Jean, is an inspiring person. Without her initial encouragement I would not have been involved in the initial breastfeeding group. I have breastfed all my children because I felt it was the natural thing to do, but never really felt the need to share my experiences with others, I thought it was something private. Once I became involved with Sure Start and Jean and began to investigate the actual benefits and amazing qualities of breastfeeding and breastmilk I discovered a passion – which has grown and grown over the last five years. I would never have envisioned being in the position that I am now. I could never have anticipated running a successful community business, employing people with the same passion and commitment as myself and the best thing, being paid to do it! I feel with Little Angels we have achieved and created a magical place where mothers can share their breastfeeding experiences and be supported through their breastfeeding career. This has only been possible with the support and help of many people who feel as passionately about breastfeeding as we do.

I feel that although breastfeeding is natural it doesn't always come naturally to all mothers and that mothers need support from other mothers.

In order to increase the breastfeeding rates in the UK, along with support, breastfeeding needs to be seen as fashionable and the norm. Little Angels aims to make breastfeeding fashionable.

I feel very proud to have been able to be part of the initiation of Little Angels and look back on what we have achieved in disbelief but also in amazement.

(Michelle Atkin)

What can midwives do?

In East Lancashire, the Little Angels model of support has brought mothers and midwives together. The initial 'suspicion' of peer support on the postnatal wards has disappeared and an environment of mutual respect and appreciation now prevails. Midwives feel delighted when a Little Angel walks on a busy postnatal ward and asks to see the mothers. The midwives are also confident that the approach and advice is consistent with theirs, they are working together to promote successful breastfeeding. It is essential that midwives make the peer supporters feel welcomed if they are all to work effectively.

Peer support is not a substitute for midwives supporting mothers to breastfeed. It is essential that maternity services ensure an environment that promotes and protects breastfeeding, by implementing an externally evaluated programme such as BFI as a minimum standard, as described above. Building on this, midwives are then in a prime position to facilitate the development of peer support programmes, to enhance the service for breastfeeding mothers, by assisting them in their role. In addition to the synthesis of 26 government-funded peer support projects Dykes (2003, 2005c) described above, Little Angels would like to offer further suggestions for midwives and health visitors to consider when working with women to establish breastfeeding peer support.

Key implications for midwifery practice

- Investigate possibility of peer support in your organisation; is there a volunteer manager in your organisation?
- Identify local mothers who successfully breastfed. You may want to liaise with health visitor colleagues. Facilitate and encourage one or two mothers taking the lead. A mother-led model of support is crucial.
- Peer support must be integrated into mainstream service from the beginning.
- Peer supporters and midwives should learn together and support each other.
- Encourage or ensure core services support and protect breastfeeding.

References

Alexander J, Anderson T, Grant M *et al.* (2003) Support group for breast-feeding women in Salisbury, UK. *Midwifery* 19: 215–20.

Anderson T, Grant M (2001) The art of community-based breastfeeding support. The Blandford breastfeeding support group, incorporating the 'Blandford Bosom Buddies'. *MIDIRS Midwifery Digest* 11(supp 1): S20–23.

Arlotti JP, Cottrell BH, Lee SH, Curtin JJ (1998) Breastfeeding among low-income women with and without peer support. *Journal of Community Health Nursing* 15: 163–78.

Barker DJP (1994) *Mothers, Babies and Disease in Later Life*. London, British Medical Journal Publications.

Battersby S (2001a) *Simply the Breast: evaluation of a peer support programme.* www.sheffield.ac.uk/surestart/brstfrnt.html (accessed 5/12/06).

Battersby S (2001b) The Worldly Wise Project: a different approach to breastfeeding support. *The Practising Midwife* 4: 30–31.

Battersby S, Sabin K (2002) Breastfeeding peer support: 'The Worldly Wise Project.' *MIDIRS Midwifery Digest* 12 (suppl 1): S29–S32.

Channel 4 *Extraordinary Breastfeeding* broadcast November 13 2006.

DeMott K, Bick D, Norman R *et al.* (2006) *Clinical Guidelines and Evidence Review for Postnatal Care: Routine postnatal care of recently delivered women and their babies*. London, National Collaborating Centre for Primary Care and Royal College of General Practitioners.

Dennis C-L (2002) Breastfeeding peer support: maternal and volunteer perceptions from a randomized controlled trial. *Birth* 29: 169–76.

Dennis C-L, Hodnett E, Gallop R, Chambers B (2002) A randomized controlled trial evaluating the effect of peer support on breastfeeding duration among primiparous women. *Canadian Medical Association Journal* 166, 21–28.

Dennis C-L (2003) Peer support within a health care context: a concept analysis. *International Journal of Nursing Studies* 40: 321–32.

Department of Health (2000): *The NHS Plan: A Plan For Investment, A Plan For Reform*. London, The Stationery Office.

Department of Health (2002) Improvement, Expansion and Reform: The Next Three Years Priorities and Planning Framework 2003–2006. www.dh.gov.uk/PublicationsAndStatistics/Publications/PublicationsPolicyAndGuidance/PublicationsPolicyAndGuidanceArticle/fs/en?CONTENT_ID=4008430&chk=lXp8vH (accessed 5/12/06).

Department of Health (2004a) *Choosing Health: Making Healthy Choices Easier*. London, The Stationery Office.

Department of Health (2005b) *Choosing a Better Diet: A Food and Health Action Plan*. London, The Stationery Office.

Dodds R (2006) Breastfeeding advice (News). *Midwives* 9(6): 222.

Dykes F, Williams C (1999) Falling by the wayside: a phenomenological exploration of perceived breast milk inadequacy in lactating women. *Midwifery* 15: 232–46.

Dykes F (2002) Western marketing and medicine: construction of an insufficient milk syndrome. *Health Care for Women International* 23: 492–502.

Dykes F (2003) Infant Feeding Initiative: *A Report Evaluating the Breastfeeding Practice Projects 1999–2002*. London, Department of Health. www.dh.gov.uk/assetRoot/04/08/44/59/04084459.pdf (accessed 5/12/06).

Dykes F (2005a) A critical ethnographic study of encounters between midwives and breast-feeding women in postnatal wards in England. *Midwifery* 21: 241–52.

Dykes F (2005b) 'Supply' and 'demand': breastfeeding as labour. *Social Science and Medicine* 60(10): 2283–93.

Dykes F (2005c) Government funded breastfeeding peer support projects: Implications for practice. *Maternal and Child Nutrition* 1: 21–31.

Dykes F, Hall Moran V (2006) Transmitted nutritional deprivation: A socio-biological perspective. In Hall Moran V, Dykes F (eds) *Maternal and Infant Nutrition and Nurture: Controversies and Challenges.* London, Quay Books.

Dykes F (2006) *Breastfeeding in Hospital: Midwives, Mothers and the Production Line.* London, Routledge.

Dyson L, Renfrew M, McFadden A *et al.* (2006) *Promotion of Breastfeeding Initiation and Duration: Evidence Into Practice Briefing.* London, National Institute for Clinical Excellence.

Haider R, Kabir I, Huttly SRA, Ashworth A (2002) Training peer counsellors to promote and support exclusive breastfeeding in Bangladesh. *Journal of Human Lactation* 18: 7–12.

Hamlyn B, Brooker S, Oleinikova K, Wands S (2002) *Infant Feeding 2000.* London, The Stationery Office.

Hawkins A, Heard S (2001) An exploration of the factors which may affect the duration of breastfeeding by first time mothers on low incomes: a multiple case study. *MIDIRS Midwifery Digest* 11: 521–26.

Health Development Agency (2004) *Social Capital for Health: issues of definition, measurement and links to health.* London, The Stationery Office.

Hoddinott P, Pill R (1999) Qualitative study of decisions about infant feeding among women in the east end of London. *British Medical Journal* 318: 30–34.

Kirkham M, Sherridan A, Thornton D, Smale M (2006) 'Breastfriends' Doncaster: the story of our peer support project. In Hall Moran V, Dykes F (eds) *Maternal and Infant Nutrition and Nurture: Controversies and Challenges.* London, Quay Books.

Kistin N, Abramson R, Dublin P (1994) Effect of peer counsellors on breastfeeding initiation: exclusivity and duration among low-income urban women. *Journal of Human Lactation* 10: 11–15.

Long DG, Funk-Archuleta MA, Gieger CJ *et al.* (1995) Peer counselor programme increases breastfeeding rates in Utah Native America WIC population. *Journal of Human Lactation* 11: 279–84.

Maternity Care Working Party (2001) *Modernising Maternity Care.* London, RCM, RCOG, NCT.

McInnes RJ, Love DH, Stone DH (2000) Evaluation of a community-based intervention to increase breastfeeding prevalence. *Journal of Public Health* 22: 138–45.

McInnes RJ, Stone DH (2001) The process of implementing a community-based peer breastfeeding support programme: the Glasgow experience. *Midwifery* 17: 65–73.

Morrow AL, Guerrero ML, Shults J *et al.* (1999) Efficacy of home-based peer counselling to promote exclusive breastfeeding: a randomised controlled trial. *Lancet* 353: 1226–1231.

Raine P, Woodward P (2003) Promoting breastfeeding: a peer support initiative. *Community Practitioner* 76: 211–14.

Sachs M (2005) *Following the Line: An ethnographic study of the influence of routine baby weighing on breastfeeding women in the North West of England.* Unpublished PhD, University of Central Lancashire.

Schafer E, Vogel MK, Viegas S, Hausafus C (1998) Volunteer peer counsellors increase breastfeeding duration among rural low-income women. *Birth* 25: 101–106.

Schmied V, Sheehan A, Barclay L (2001) Contemporary Breastfeeding Policy and Practice: implications for midwives. *Midwifery* 17: 44–54.

Scott J, Mostyn T (2003) Women's experiences of breastfeeding in a bottle feeding culture. *Journal of Human Lactation* 19: 270–77.

Sellen DW (2001) Weaning, complementary feeding, and maternal decision making in a rural East African pastoral population. *Journal of Human Lactation* 17: 233–44.

Shaw E, Kaczorowski J (1999) The effect of a peer counseling program on breastfeeding initiation and longevity in a low-income rural population. *Journal of Human Lactation* 15: 19–25.

Smale M (2004) *Training Breastfeeding Peer Supporters: An Enabling Approach.* Women's Informed Childbearing and Health (WICH) Research group. University of Sheffield Publication (Obtainable from v.mathers@sheffield.ac.uk).

Sookhoo M, King A, Gibb C (2002) Evaluating breastfeeding support by lay support workers in an area of the UK with low breastfeeding success rates. *International Confederation of Midwives Triennial Congress*, Vienna, Austria, 2002. Proceedings CD-ROM, Austria, Marshall.

Timms M (2002) What are Osmaston and Allenton Sure Start doing towards community based breastfeeding support? A midwife's story. *MIDIRS Midwifery Digest* 12: 278–79.

UNICEF Baby Friendly Initiative website: www.babyfriendly.org.uk/ (accessed 6/12/06).

Wright J (1996) Breastfeeding and deprivation: the Nottingham peer counsellor programme. *MIDIRS Midwifery Digest* 6: 212–15.

Wright AL, Naylor A, Wester R, Bauer M, Sutcliffe E (1997) Using cultural knowledge in health promotion: breastfeeding among the Navajo. *Health Education and Behaviour* 24: 625–39.

Notes

1 A unitary authority is a type of local authority, which has a single tier and is responsible for all local government functions within its area.

This is as opposed to a two-tier system where local government functions are divided between different authorities.

2 TrusTECH funding. TrusTECH is the North West NHS Innovation Hub. The hub is a partnership project set up to help NHS Trusts to manage the outputs of publicly funded research to improve healthcare. See www.trustech.org.uk/

Chapter 10
Normal Birth and Birth Centre Care: A Public Health Catalyst for Maternal and Societal Well-being

Soo Downe and Denis Walsh

> I have stated on numerous occasions that there is no more need to interfere with the course of normally progressing labour than there is to tamper with good digestion, normal respiration and adequate circulation
>
> (Montgomery 1958)

Introduction

The term 'normal' to describe labour and childbirth has been in common use for centuries. However, the vast body of research in the field of maternity services is centred on potential problems or pathologies. Recent research has demonstrated that few births recorded as 'normal spontaneous delivery' take place without a series of technological interventions (Downe *et al.* 2001, Mead 2004). As other authors in this book have indicated, the concept of 'public health' is more recent. It has undergone a transformation in the Western world from its initial concentration on hygiene and public sanitation, to current so-called 'lifestylism' and, at the extreme, the criminalisation of individuals who transgress medically mediated norms of good public health behaviour (Cahill 1999).

New ways of constructing both childbirth and public health are explored in this final chapter, as a focus for further thinking. Two examples are given to illustrate these, one from Brazil which engages with a fresh understanding of the role of childbirth in the local community's health; and the other from the UK which examines the impact of the birth centre model on healthcare staff and women users. The potential consequences of a new vision of child-birth and the changed organisational models to support it are clin-ical, psychological, and societal. A turn away from pathology and towards well-being is proposed, based on the concepts of unique normality, salutogenesis, complexity and uncertainty (Downe 2006). Alongside this, new models of provision are required to reflect these values. In keeping with the philosophy of this book, the chapter proposes that all midwives can use this way of seeing with each individual woman they encounter, to increase overall public health.

Background

Current definitions of 'normal childbirth' range from the purely clinical (WHO 1997) to the transformational (Bennett and Brown 1993, Royal College of Midwives (RCM) 1997; Downe and McCourt 2004). In the late 1990s, there were a number of reports on the subject of normal birth from official bodies (Clinical Standards Advisory Group 1995; World Health Organization 1997, RCM 1997); and the recent *National Framework for Children, Young People, and Maternity* (DoH 2004) re-emphasises the need to maximise spontaneous birth where possible. The nature of normality expressed in these reports varies considerably. Williams and col-leagues report an intrapartum survey of primigravid women in England and Scotland, which records unexpectedly high levels of intervention (Williams *et al.* 1998). A subsequent regional study of the incidence of intervention in normal labour which found that only 1:4 of all primigravid women, and fewer than 1:3 multigravid women, experienced spontaneous vaginal birth without at least one of five prespecified interventions, namely induction or aug-mentation of labour, episiotomy, epidural analgesia, or artificial rupture of membranes (Downe *et al.* 2001; Beech 1997). More recently, Marianne Mead concluded from a survey of practice in 11 maternity units that midwives in her study tended to approach birth as 'a catastrophe waiting to happen' (Mead 2004:80).

Clinically, the most obvious implication of current ways of doing birth is an apparently inexorable rise in rates of caesarean section. Although maternal mortality associated with elective caesarean section has fallen dramatically, possible adverse mater-nal and neonatal consequences remain. These include secondary infertility (Murphy *et al.* 2002); higher risk of stillbirth in sub-sequent pregnancies (Smith *et al.* 2003); and newly emerging indications that mode of birth affects neonatal immune system adjustment (Grönlund *et al.* 1999). The evidence is mixed on postnatal depression, but, in individual cases, incidences of maternal unhappiness are evidenced following normal birth with interventions as well as surgical births (Beech and Phipps 2004). These technologic ways of birthing also appear to result in higher costs (Petrou and Glazener 2002), higher rates of attrition of midwives (Ball *et al.* 2002) and much higher rates of litigation.

Public health is currently of increasing concern to governments and to public bodies. While the genesis of this concern probably arose in the 19th century, the following statement from the World Health Organization captures the generally accepted intent of current public health endeavours:

Health is . . .

. . . a complete state of physical, mental and social well-being and not merely the absence of disease or infirmity
(World Health Organization 1948)

In parallel with changes in concepts of 'normal' birth, constructions of public health have undergone a transformation in the Western world, from an initial concentration on hygiene and public sanitation, to current so-called 'lifestylism', which focuses on acceptable or unacceptable lifestyle choices of individuals based on population-wide evidence. As noted above, at the extreme, this approach leads to the criminalisation of those who transgress medically mediated norms of good public health behaviour (Skrabanek 1994; Cahill 1999). In the context of childbirth, a healthism stance may involve a greater risk of interventions forced on the mother or parents, in opposition to their choices. This has resulted in court-ordered caesarean section in the UK and America, court-ordered use of formula milk for a breastfed baby whose mother was HIV-positive, and enforced measles-mumps-rubella (MMR) immunisation of two children after the estranged fathers brought a legal case against the mothers who genuinely feared damage to their children if the immunisation went ahead (Anon 2003). Such outcomes result from a public health driven by targets and population-based evidence.

A new way of seeing

It may be that a change of emphasis is needed in the way childbirth is understood. This may also have resonance for the kind of public health that holds sway. We have examined the current childbirth paradigm in some detail (Downe and McCourt 2004). We have proposed that childbirth (and most Western medicine) is framed in pathology, simplicity and certainty. We suggest that childbirth can be reframed on the basis of three approaches:

- Salutogenesis (or the generation of well-being, Antonovsky 1987)
- Complexity
- Uncertainty.

Following Davis-Floyd and Davis (1997) we stated:

> In this construction, each woman's labour is unique to her and her baby, and to the interaction and connectivity between her personal and familial history, the environment in which she labours, the attitude and response of the caregiver(s), and to a multitude of other factors
>
> (Downe and McCourt 2004)

The characteristics of 'unique normality' thinking lead practitioners to see birth as dynamic and unpredictable, with the clinical safety of mother and baby the absolute minimum requirement, rather than the primary focus. Practitioners who approach each woman's birth as an event that is uniquely normal for her seem to see the process as catalytic and potentially transformational rather than purely physical (Davis-Floyd and Davis 1997). This way of seeing allows for the possibility of emergence, or for the unexpected, both at an individual and societal level. From a public health perspective, it recognises that there is a connection between healthy individuals and healthy societies, but that the direction of this emergent well-being may not be possible to predict, or to engineer. Do healthy individuals create healthy societies, or vice versa? The relevant public health framework is probably that given in Donaldson and Donaldson (2000), based on criteria from the WHO European Region Healthy Cities project:

- Building public health policy
- Creating supportive environments
- Strengthening community action
- Developing personal skills
- Reorientating health services

Donaldson and Donaldson (2000:116)

Examples of good practice: Project Luz

There are examples of personal and societal well-being arising from systems of childbirth that maximise the potential of positive birthing. For example, Belinda Phipps explores the implications through women's stories, including the following (Phipps 2002):

> My personal experience really makes me believe that birth matters and has implications throughout the child's life
>
> The way a woman gives birth can affect the whole of the rest of her life – how can that not matter? Unless the woman herself doesn't matter
>
> Beech and Phipps give examples of how, for some women, birth experiences resonate into their relationships with their children over many years (Beech and Phipps 2004).

A clear example of the societal impact of positive birthing is that of Project Luz (Misago *et al.* 2001. This project was based in Brazil, where there have historically been very high rates of caesarean section. Childbirth in Brazil, as in many countries, has been heavily influenced by the widescale exportation of technocratic and interventionist ways of doing birth. In many of these settings, women labour together with minimal privacy and social support in cold or overheated labour rooms, and experience routine interventions such as enemas and augmentation of labour (El-Nemer *et al.* 2005). The researchers running the project started by asking local men and women in five municipalities in north-east Brazil a number of questions. These included their perception of health priorities for the local community (Misago *et al.* 2001). Childhood diarrhoea was at the top of the list of these priorities. Women's issues, and, specifically, childbirth, hardly featured.

The researchers then spent the next three years 'humanising' birth in these locations. This involved simple actions, such as ensuring companionship and some degree of privacy for labouring women. After the project the researchers went back to ask representatives of the local community what the most important health issues were. As the researchers say, 'comments such as "normal vaginal delivery is best for women and babies" became frequently heard among men and women in the community'. A clue as to why this was is given in the following comment from one of the researchers:

> Project Luz has given many women the feeling of strong confidence in a safe delivery and in child rearing . . . leading to self-transformation, which empowers them profoundly. This . . . raises their concerns about society, their lives, and motivates their participation in community activities and development
>
> (Umenai 2001)

In this case, the impact of an approach that sought to maximise women's well-being during labour and birth had an impact beyond the individual woman. It extended into a transformational view of both personal and the wider public health. The emergent impact was unlooked for, but very powerful.

While this may be interesting, it could be argued that it does not have immediate resonance for the resource-rich countries of the West. The debate around place of birth offers a parallel example for childbirth-related public health in resource-rich countries. The issue of place of birth is usually discussed in the context of safety. In contrast, we would like to explore it to illustrate how the provision of alternative settings for birth may increase public health and societal well-being, both for those using the service, and for those working within it, through strong idealistic identification, and subsequent local and political lobbying.

Examples in practice: UK freestanding birth centres

Freestanding birth centres, formally known as isolated general practitioner maternity units, have always represented a wellness model because they offer facilities where the emphasis is on an expectation that birth will go well, and on supportive midwifery care. More recently, they have demonstrated community empowerment through resisting closure pressures coming from acute hospital trusts and strategic health authorities. Over the past three decades their numbers have reduced from in the hundreds in the 1970s (Young 1987) to fewer than 80 in 2002 (Duerden 2001). Reasons for closure ranged from traditional concerns about safety, through to their cost, and finally to the perception that they were chronically underused.

In the last five years, other driving forces have paradoxically led to their steady increase. First, the rationalisation of neonatal facilities has led to the closure of small consultant maternity units, which have become midwifery-led units or birth centres. Second, local opposition has led to the forestalling of some planned closures and the fresh opening of new facilities. It is this latter trend that we will expand on here because it represents genuine community empowerment. In a number of places around the UK, local campaigns have successfully overturned bureaucratic decisions and many of their stories have made the news headlines nationally (Boseley 2006). They often seem to be an alliance of midwives, local childbearing women, general practitioners and local politicians who successfully fight institutional and bureaucratic forces in David-versus-Goliath-style struggles. Denis Walsh explores this in the next section, based on his recent ethnographic study of a birth centre.

My own research (DW) discovered this in a birth centre in the midlands of England where closure was planned at the end of the 1990s. A steering group consisting of midwives, local women and a GP ran a campaign over a 12-month period that eventually secured the future of the centre. They became adept at lobbying and campaigning skills and gave an enormous amount of time outside work hours to the cause. They were fighting to retain local birthing, which had been present in the community since the Second World War. As the birth centre staff told me, it was their livelihood and their way of life now under threat that motivated them. The skills they learnt over this time have been mirrored in other struggles for retaining local birth facilities and include:

- Using media
- Using influential others
- Using public opinion
- Assertiveness
- Delegation/organisation.

The success of the campaign had a profound effect on both the staff at the birth centre and the women users, captured in this statement by one of the midwives:

> I really wouldn't mind having a go at anything. That's not how I was a few years ago! But now because of the unit being under threat of closure, it's another dimension! We've really grown here. I don't want to sound arrogant, but I am important, I am doing things, I am making a difference

When I interviewed women, some could not understand me asking a question about why they chose to have their baby at the birth centre. As one woman said: 'I was born here. So were my brothers and sisters. Why would I want to go anywhere else?' There was a definite sense of the birth centre having been part of the community for generations. One of the key moments in the campaign was the rally in the town centre to which the media were invited. Thousands of families turned up so that traffic was brought to a standstill and the media coverage extensive. Ten thousand petition signatures were collected and presented to the local Member of Parliament. This was community empowerment at its most effective and tangible. It provides encouragement to other maternity services in the country that are being reconfigured against the wishes of local staff and populations.

Maternity care viewed as a public health issue can motivate communities to fight for local birthing provision. Birth centre services also challenge the dominant model of clinical care. This is the biomedical technocratic model, premised on reducing mortality and morbidity. Research into women's preference for birth centre care suggests that, in contrast, a social model (Walsh and Newburn 2002) dominates their thinking. The language used by women in my study indicated this, as they described the birth centre as a 'B and B', a 'small hotel', a 'health spa', 'my bedroom'. It as if they were deliberately distinguishing the facility from a hospital. They spoke of it being a baby-friendly place, welcoming, peaceful and calm. They felt at ease and at home there, contrasting this with previous negative experiences in hospitals where care was rushed, impersonal and clinical. They spoke at length about the décor, ambience and nurturing environment they found there. Staff concerns about 'making over' the birth rooms reflected their concern with this environmental aspect and I theorised that both women and staff were expressing a kind of 'nesting' instinct (Walsh 2006b). I believe this was grounded in the mammalian instinct to protect their offspring from intruders, from environmental hazards and from predators. Women were reframing safety to incorporate psychological, social and cultural safety in a deliberate turn away from a purely biomedical understanding of safety.

This embracing of a social model of care resonates with salutogenesis and well-being (Downe and McCourt 2004). The birth centre demonstrates this in the very low intervention rates during labour and birth. In effect, local maternity care is aligned with a public health model of childbirth as integral to the local community and experienced as a 'rites of passage' transition that is person and family-centred, not an event orchestrated by professionals.

Another aspect of birth centre work, a serendipitous finding that was not expected, links to community empowerment and capacity-building. Though this is principally mediated by the staff for the staff, it has knock-on effects for the women and their families. This was the considerable store of social capital found in the setting. Interviews revealed the sense of job fulfilment and belonging that staff had for the centre, typified by the following remark from a midwife:

> Working here is like having your favourite chocolate bar. You really want it, you get to have it and you still want some more. It's lovely

Conditions that contributed to this were part-time hours, flexible shift patterns, reciprocal childcare arrangements, a blurring of work/life boundaries, support through personal crises and an established pattern of social outings. All of these were supported by a sympathetic manager.

Social capital theory can be defined as:

> the networks, norms, relationships, values and informal sanctions that shape the quantity and co-operative quality of a society's social interactions
>
> (Aldridge *et al.* 2002)

It is premised on trust, high levels of volunteerism and participation (Knack and Keefer 2000). There are a number of common threads between the theory of social capital and the internal and external dynamics of the birth centre in this study. The first is to do with 'community'. At the heart of community is the sense of belonging and commitment to each other. These often cluster around a shared identity. Edmondson (2003) cites examples of how social capital builds up in communities exposed to threat. Parallels are clear with recent birth centre history. In the late 1990s, an alignment of staff and consumers resisted health authority efforts to close down the unit I was studying. The solidarity of struggle was identity-shaping for staff at the centre, and reinforced an existing sense of belonging cultivated by the lead midwife appointed in 1993. The attributes of identity and belonging led to both reciprocal and non-reciprocal giving. This reciprocity was apparent in the working lives of staff at the birth centre where flexibility with work patterns was endemic. Non-reciprocal giving was manifest in the amount of birth centre activity that took place in the staff's own time, be that fundraising, meetings and support for individuals in crisis through phone calls or visiting.

Staff willingness to volunteer for activities, and to participate in the life of the birth centre stood out as further indicators of social capital. Though levels of participation varied, nobody, it seemed, was outside of the loop. Everybody went to at least some of the monthly social outings; everybody contributed in some way to maintaining and improving the upkeep of the centre and to fundraising events.

Finally, trust is considered a cornerstone of social capital. It operates at an individual level between group members, at a social level between members and outsiders, and at a hierarchical level in relation to the governance of formal institutions.

The birth centre exuded trust at an individual level, in part facilitated not just by work relationships, but also by friend relationships among the staff. Compassionate responses to personal problems were one manifestation of this. Longevity of employment seemed to play a part in cultivating mutual understanding and tolerance to the mix of personalities. Trust of the women entering the birth centre was also high, as demonstrated by the accommodation of women's choices for their labour and postnatal care (Walsh 2006a).

Many of the characteristics of work-life at the birth centre that contributed to social capital stemmed from economies of scale. Scale affects time management, providing space to build strong interpersonal relationships among staff. Meaningful relationships become unrealistic as the number of people in a social grouping increase. Once numbers grow beyond a workable team ethos, then there is a need for structural investment in social capital. Larger maternity units, if they are to replicate the advantages of social capital demonstrated here, will have to make this structural investment by, for example, devolving responsibilities to self-managing teams.

This aspect of the life of the birth centre was an unexpected and serendipitous finding. It offers promise to maternity services struggling with recruitment and retention problems. Here were maternity care staff who were not only fulfilled in their work, but who had also generated social capital that would compare favourably with many voluntary organisations.

Example of good practice: Brisbane, Australia

- In Brisbane, Australia, a birth centre attached to a large metropolitan hospital, took the initiative to explore a user forum of women who had used the centre.
- To their surprise, they were overwhelmed with interest from women and within two months, a Friends of the Birth Centre Group had formed.
- They meet monthly with the midwives with a remit for mutual support and fundraising for the centre.
- Now three years later, they have a proactive role in evolving the service with representatives on strategy groups within the hospital and publish a bimonthly Newsletter that is distributed throughout other maternity user groups in Queensland.

Conclusion

Changing our way of seeing childbirth, and therefore of the way we respond to women, may also change the way we think about and create public health. If current constructions of childbirth can be reoriented from a pathological, simplistic, certainty way of thinking to one founded in unique normality thinking, the public health consequences may be far reaching. As Kitzinger (1987) states:

> To anyone who thinks about it long enough, birth cannot simply be a matter of techniques for getting a baby out of one's body. It involves our relationship to life as a whole, the part we play in the order of things
>
> Kitzinger (1987)

Changing the way we work together can address the health and wholeness of staff, which will also have effects for health, and for the happiness of women in our care. This has been demonstrated by both the La Paz example, and the by the case of the freestanding birth centre model described above. Through a shared solidarity in the face of adversity, both schemes evolved a social model of care that had, as a knock-on effect, the generation of considerable social capital. These models challenge maternity units to replicate aspects of care that may bring about similar effects, potentially addressing both safe motherhood issues, and iatrogenic intervention in childbirth, and softening the institutionalising and dehumanising face of hospital bureaucracy.

Key implications for midwifery practice

- The way women experience pregnancy and childbirth can be catalytic for their self-perception and for the way they relate to their family and their society.
- This effect can be positive or negative for personal and public health.
- Every caregiver has the potential to positively influence individual and public health for each woman, baby, and family they meet.
- To maximise the potential for well-being, after each appointment or birth, midwives could ask 'did this woman leave my care feeling better about herself than before I met her?'
- Public health can benefit from population led and pathology driven initiatives, but it can also emerge from individual encounters based on the promotion of well-being and tailored to meet the complexity of individual lives.

References

Aldridge S, Halpern D, Fitzpatrick S (2002) *Social Capital: A Discussion Paper*. London, Performance and Innovation Unit.

Anon (2003) Court orders girls to have MMR jab. *Guardian Unlimited* June 13. www.guardian.co.uk/medicine/story/0,11381,977145,00.html (accessed 6/12/06).

Antonovsky A (1987) *Unravelling the Mystery of Health: How People Manage Stress and Stay Well*. San Francisco, CA, Jossey-Bass.

Ball L, Curtis P, Kirkham M (2002) *Why Do Midwives Leave?* Available from: The Royal College of Midwives, RCM Publications Office, UK Board for Wales, 4 Cathedral Road, Cardiff, CF11 9LJ.

Beech BAL (1997) Normal birth – does it exist? *Association for Improvements in the Maternity Services Journal* 9(2): 4–8.

Beech BL, Phipps B (2004) Normal birth: women's stories. In Downe S (ed) *Normal Birth: Evidence and Debate*. Oxford, Elsevier.

Bennett VR, Brown LK (1993) *Myles Textbook for Midwives*. Edinburgh, Churchill Livingstone, p 149.

Boseley S (2006) Midwife-led birth centres threatened by cost cutting. *The Guardian* May 20, 2006 http://society.guardian.co.uk/publicfinances/story/0,,1780458,00.html (accessed 6/12/06).

Cahill H (1999) An Orwellian scenario: court-ordered caesarean section and women's autonomy. *Nursing Ethics* 6(6): 494–505.

Chirico G, Gasparoni A, Ciardelli L *et al.* (1999) Leukocyte counts in relation to the method of delivery during the first five days of life. *Biology of the Neonate* 75(5): 294–99.

Clinical Standards Advisory Group (1995) *Women in Normal Labour*. London, HMSO.

Davis-Floyd R, Davis E (1997) Intuition as authoritative knowledge in midwifery and home birth. In Davis-Floyd R and Arvidson PS (eds) *Intuition: The Inside Story: Interdisciplinary Perspectives*. New York, Routledge.

Department of Health (2004) *National Service Framework for children, young people and maternity services*. London, The Stationery Office.

Donaldson LJ, Donaldson RJ (2000) *Essential Public Health* (2nd edn). Newbury, Petroc Press.

Downe S (2006) Engaging with the concept of unique normality in childbirth. *British Journal of Midwifery* 14(6): 352–56.

Downe S, McCormick C, Beech B (2001) Labour interventions associated with normal birth. *British Journal of Midwifery* 9 (10): 602–606.

Downe S, McCourt C (2004) From being to becoming: reconstructing childbirth knowledges. In Downe S (ed) *Normal Birth: evidence and debate*. Oxford, Elsevier.

Duerden J (2001) *Directory of Freestanding Low Risk Maternity Units in England*. Leeds, Yorkshire Consortium of Local Supervising Authorities.

Edmondson R (2003) Social Capital: a strategy for enhancing health. *Social Science and Medicine* 57: 1723–33.

El-Nemer A, Downe S, Small N (2005) She would help me from the heart: an ethnography of Egyptian women in labour. *Social Science and Medicine* 62(1): 81–92.

Grönlund MM, Nuutila J, Pelto L *et al.* (1999) Mode of delivery directs the phagocyte functions of infants for the first 6 months of life. *Clinical and Experimental Immunology* 116: 521–26.

Kitzinger S (1987) *Freedom and Choice In Childbirth.* Harmondsworth, Viking.

Knack S, Keefer P (2000) Does social capital have an economic payoff? *Quarterly Journal of Economics* 112: 1251–85.

Mead M (2004) Midwives practice in 11 UK maternity units. In Downe S (ed) *Normal Birth: evidence and debate.* Oxford, Elsevier.

Misago C, Kendall C, Freitas P *et al.* (2001) From 'culture of dehumanization of childbirth' to 'childbirth as a transformative experience': changes in five municipalities in north-east Brazil. *International Journal of Gynecology and Obstetrics* 75: S67–S72.

Montgomery TL (1958) Physiological considerations in labor and the puerperium. *American Journal of Obstetrics and Gynecology* 76: 706–15.

Murphy DJ, Stirrat GM, Heron J and Alspac Study Team (2002) The relationship between caesarean section and subfertility in a population-based sample of 14 541 pregnancies. *Human Reproduction* 17(7): 1914–17.

Petrou S, Glazener C (2002) The economic costs of alternative modes of delivery during the first two months postpartum: results from a Scottish observational study. *British Journal of Obstetrics and Gynaecology* 109(2): 214–17.

Phipps B (2002) Normal birth – does it matter? *The Practising Midwife* 5(2): 23–24.

Royal College Of Midwives (1997) *Debating Midwifery: Normality in Midwifery.* London, RCM.

Skrabanek P (1994) *The Death of Humane Medicine and the Rise of Coercive Healthism.* Bury St Edmunds, Social Affairs Unit, St Edmundsbury Press.

Smith GC, Pell JP, Dobbie R (2003) Caesarean section and risk of unexplained stillbirth in subsequent pregnancy. *Lancet* 362: 1779–84.

Umenai T (2001) Forewords of the International Conference on the Humanization of Childbirth. *International Journal of Gynaecology and Obstetrics* 75: S1–S2.

Walsh D, Newburn M (2002) Towards a social model of childbirth: part 1. *British Journal of Midwifery* 10(8): 476–81.

Walsh D (2006a) Subverting assembly-line birth: Childbirth in a free-standing birth centre. *Social Science and Medicine* 62(6): 1330–40.

Walsh D (2006b) 'Nesting' and 'Matrescence': Distinctive Features of a Free-Standing Birth Centre. *Midwifery* 22(3): 228–39.

Williams FL, Florey CV, Ogston SA *et al.* (1998) UK study of intrapartum care for low risk primigravidas: a survey of interventions. *Journal of Epidemiology and Community Health* 52(8): 494–500.

World Health Organization (1948) *Constitution: Basic Documents.* Geneva, WHO.

World Health Organization Department of Reproductive Health and Research (1997) Care in normal birth: a practical guide. Geneva, WHO.

Young G (1987) Are isolated maternity units run by general practitioners dangerous? *British Medical Journal* 294: 744–46.

Index

05098569

Lightning Source UK Ltd.
Milton Keynes UK
UKOW042147290212

188081UK00004B/14/P